D1327336

Five Constraints on Predicting Behavior

Five Constraints on Predicting Behavior

Jerome Kagan

The MIT Press
Cambridge, Massachusetts
London, England

This book was set in ITC Stone Sans Std and ITC Stone Serif Std by Toppan Best-set Premedia Limited. Printed and bound in the United States of America.

Library of Congress Cataloging-in-Publication Data

Names: Kagan, Jerome, author.
Title: Five constraints on predicting behavior / Jerome Kagan.
Description: Cambridge, MA : MIT Press, [2017] | Includes bibliographical references and index.
Identifiers: LCCN 2016055174 | ISBN 9780262036528 (hardcover : alk. paper)
Subjects: LCSH: Human behavior. | Psychology. | Neuropsychology.
Classification: LCC BF199 .K234 2017 | DDC 150--dc23 LC record available at https://lccn.loc.gov/2016055174

10 9 8 7 6 5 4 3 2 1

Contents

Preface

The anthropologist Loren Eiseley divided scientists into little- and big-bone hunters. The latter ask the profound questions that require more effort but rouse the curiosity of minds that wonder why this way rather than that. Five questions have always been high on the list of puzzles. How did the universe form? How did life emerge? Why does like beget like? Why do living forms die? What processes allow a person to perceive, remember, infer, reason, feel, and act?

The happy wedding of human imagination and elegant machines provided preliminary answers to the first four questions, allowing the fifth to ascend in the hierarchy of puzzling phenomena considered amenable to solution.

The study of brain–mind relations had to wait for the invention of technologies that could measure the brain activity accompanying psychological processes that were not apparent in observable behavior. Alfred North Whitehead, reflecting on the discoveries of the quantum revolution, commented that the physicists responsible for these victories were not smarter than their nineteenth-century mentors. They had the advantage of better machines.

Because the technology available to contemporary students of the brain still cannot measure the rapidly changing sequence of phenomena that precedes a psychological outcome, most conclusions remain tentative. Some are simply wrong. This essay considers five conditions that constrain confident inferences about the relation between brain profiles and a variety of psychological phenomena. They are the influence of the context on the evidence gathered; the expectations of the participants; the source of evidence for an inference; the habit of looking for relations between single causes and single outcomes; and the attribution of psychological concepts to brain patterns.

Although I spent my research career trying to understand aspects of the psychological development of children, I tried meanwhile to keep abreast of the work in neuroscience. One of the gifts of retirement was the opportunity to spend uninterrupted hours reading the relevant literature. An earlier book, *A Young Mind in a Growing Brain* (Kagan & Herschkowitz, 2005), summarized what was known about the relation between the maturation of the human brain and the development of psychological properties during the child's first decade. The purpose of this slimmer volume is to prod the scientists and students who labor in the territory of mind-brain relations to reflect on the currently popular collection of beliefs and to consider adopting some of the practices I advocate.

Illumination of the events that make psychological phenomena possible will benefit many constituencies, while bringing immense satisfaction to those responsible for the insights. I hope this discussion of the factors that constrain current generalizations is of some help to the brilliant scientists engaged in this mission.

1 Introduction

Scientists interested in understanding the psychological properties of adult humans have replaced an earlier emphasis on the
role of experience with a search for correspondences between
brain profiles and a psychological outcome. Although the new
paradigm is young, the inability to understand the brain states
that generate most mental events, along with the actions that
may follow, frustrates scientists and disappoints those who
support them. Although physicists massage the egos of those
engaged in this endeavor by confessing that the brain is far
more complex than atoms, the sparseness of headline-grabbing
victories that go unchallenged remains a troubling irritant. The
culprits are insensitive methods, weak theories, and inadequate
funding for younger investigators. This book examines five additional reasons for a pace of progress that is slower than earlier
generations anticipated.

For most of human history a person's beliefs about nature,
society, and the self's properties were based on personal experiences, conversations with others, and pronouncements by
respected authorities. The first source of information necessarily
occurred in a specific context; the latter two typically implied
a context. A friend telling another about the dangers of a food,

animal, or stranger usually contextualizes the threat in sentences such as, "There is a new wolf in the vicinity," or "The man who came to the village last month stole some corn from a neighbor." New sources of information—initially telescopes, microscopes, air pumps, thermometers, and clocks, and later the complex machines of physics, chemistry, and biology—provided novel evidence, described with a special vocabulary, that challenged the validity of traditional beliefs based on experience and hearsay. The public does not always appreciate that the validity of expert opinions, on topics ranging from health and crime to the age of the universe and the origin of life, is dependent on particular classes of evidence.

Natural scientists have learned that the validity of many if not most inferences is limited to the conditions under which the observations were gathered, until someone demonstrates their generality. For reasons that are difficult to understand, some psychologists and neuroscientists fail to attribute sufficient power to the context of observation. The second chapter considers the diverse ways in which the setting constrains the conclusions extracted from observations on one sample observed in one place with one procedure.

The context includes not only the physical and social features of the place where data are collected, but also the procedure, the collection of incentives presented, and the species, age, and sex of both the subjects and the examiner. When the subjects are humans, the language used to communicate with them is part of the context. Each context is associated with a set of probabilities assigned to the collection of likely outcomes. The context selects one response from a larger set of possible alternatives to that incentive.

The habit of underestimating the influence of the setting is due, partly, to the fact that English-speaking scientists have, up to now, performed most of the research on the brain and its relation to behavior. Most English predicates for brain processes or behaviors contain no information about the context. Verbs such as *compute, regulate,* and *integrate* provide no clue to the setting in which the process occurred. This is not true of all languages. The Japanese use different verbs to describe a person crossing an open space that is free of objects and one crossing a space that contains a railroad track, fallen logs, or boulders.

Neighborhoods, regions, nations, and cultures during particular historical eras present their residents with distinctive settings that invite a limited set of responses while making it difficult to implement others. Many of the mental illness categories in the psychiatrist's diagnostic manual describe symptoms that local circumstances made easier to acquire. Societies that offer no opportunities for gambling will have few patients with gambling disorder. There are few cases of substance abuse in cultures free of alcohol, cocaine, and opioids. The critic Arthur Danto (2009) recognized the influence of the setting on the judgment of some objects as works of art. No contemporary adult who saw a porcelain urinal, a metal tree, or a pile of tires in a hardware store would classify it as a work of art but might do so in the gallery of a modern art museum.

The circumstances in a particular society, especially its class structure, economy, ethnic diversity, and population density affect many traits. It is not a coincidence that the rise in complaints of loneliness among Americans and Europeans over the past 50 years tracks the increase in the proportion of the population living in an urban setting.

The subject's expectations comprise a second constraint on inferences. Although the events anticipated always depend on the context, this limitation is considered separately in chapter 3. Volunteers for a psychological experiment on the brain and emotion do not expect the friendly examiner to show them pictures of angry faces, snakes, guns, or bloodied bodies. The resulting activation of the amygdala is a sign of surprise rather than a reflection of fear or anxiety. Had the examiner told the participants what they would see, the amygdalar response would have been muted. Rats expect neither the sudden onset of tone nor the tingle of an electric shock to the paws that follows. Their behavioral and biological reactions are potentiated by the unexpectedness of these events, and are muted when they can anticipate the sequence.

The participants in Stanley Milgram's (1974) famous studies of conformity to authority held the expectation that an examiner employed by a respected university would not ask them to inflict serious harm on another person. Hence, they were willing to administer strong shocks to a stranger who simulated pain. The workers at Nazi concentration camps did not hold the same belief about the intentions of the high-ranking officers who told them to gas, shoot, or torture prisoners. Therefore, it is not obvious that the actions of Milgram's volunteers help us understand their behaviors.

The brain continually primes the neurons that normally respond to the event that is expected to occur in the next moment. This preparation facilitates its detection. Usually, the event anticipated is the one that occurs. On the less frequent occasions when the expectation is violated, the brain responds. Every brain profile, therefore, is a blend of the response to the event in the perceptual field and the response to the event that was anticipated. If the latter does not occur, the brain's response to the violation of expectation becomes part of the reaction to the event that occurs. This fact constrains inferences about psychological states that are based on brain reactions to unexpected events gathered on human subjects lying supine in a magnetic scanner in an unfamiliar laboratory room.

Expectations affect many phenomena. Adults who display traits or actions that violate community expectations are likely to be rejected or victimized. Most youngsters who are bullied possess features that deviate from those expected by a majority of their peers. They might be poor, speak with a foreign dialect, have difficulty mastering the academic courses, be burdened with a physical disability, or fail to conform to the peer group's code on proper sex role behavior. Patients in psychotherapy attribute special curative power to rituals in the treatment process that are unexpected, on the assumption that a new form of treatment is likely to be better than a familiar one.

Humans prefer to spend their days in a narrow space, bordered on the left by boredom with the overly familiar and on the right by the terror of chronic unpredictability. Dictators exploit this uncomfortable state by replacing the lack of predictability that leads to civil unrest with greater certainty. Most humans living in chaotic communities are willing to give up their personal freedom in exchange for more predictable moments.

A large number of investigators studying brain–behavior relations resist Niels Bohr's insight that the validity of every conclusion is depends on its source of evidence. Two statements referring to the same observation can have dissimilar validities if they originated in different kinds of evidence. Isaac Newton relied on the text in Revelation, the last book of the Bible, to predict that the world would last until 2060. Even though this prediction is likely to be affirmed, its validity differs from the validity of the same declaration by contemporary scientists using observations from space telescopes. The validity of Lamarck's claim that an animal's experiences can alter its genome differs from the validity of an identical claim by a geneticist who is relying on epigenetic marks.

The validity of statements about security of attachment that are based on the behaviors of one-year-olds in Mary Ainsworth's Strange Situation is not the same as the validity of conclusions drawn from the verbal narratives of adults recalling their childhood. Declarations about a person's understanding of the concept of number that rely on activation of the intraparietal sulcus in the parietal lobe while subjects are discriminating between arrays of black dots have a validity that is distinct from the validity of conclusions derived from successful performance on arithmetic problems. The validity of estimates of the heritability of intelligence based on equations whose values were the degree of behavioral similarity among the biologically related members of a family does not correspond to the validity of the considerably smaller estimates derived from similarity in genomes.

One reason why brain and psychological data yield conclusions with differing validities is that some brain measures are subject to the effects of bodily processes that exert minimal effects on many psychological observations. A majority of conclusions regarding the contribution of brain states to human psychological states are based on changes in deoxygenated hemoglobin that give rise to the BOLD signal in adults lying still and supine in the narrow tube of a MRI scanner. In this setting the person's posture, breathing, and cardiovascular dynamics exert a nontrivial influence on the evidence.

Adults who award a privileged validity to conclusions about psychological outcomes that contain brain data do not extend this preference for reductive accounts to all statements in physics or biology. The immaterial nature of mental phenomena sustains the bias. Many find it more satisfying to read, "Youth who commit violent crimes are likely to possess immature frontal lobes" than to read, "Youth who commit violent crimes are likely to have grown up in families that did not socialize the restraint of asocial actions." But these same individuals do not find the sentence "The uncontrolled movements of patients with Huntington's disease are due to an abnormal gene" less satisfying than "The uncontrolled movements of patients with Huntington's disease are due to an abnormal pattern of atoms in a select sequence of nucleotides."

Many social scientists continue to rely only on a person's verbal reports of their traits or past experiences as the basis for bold conclusions about behavior or mood, even though the correspondence between these reports and direct observations is often poor. The claim that there are five major personality dimensions—agreeableness, conscientiousness, extraversion, openness to ideas, and neuroticism—the so-called Big Five—based on answers to a questionnaire, has a special validity. Different, but not less important, personality dimensions would emerge from behavioral observations.

The psychologists active before the Second World War recognized the poor correspondence between what people said about themselves or their past and other sources of information. Many hoped that interpretations given to Rorschach inkblots and scenes in the Thematic Apperception Test would reveal more accurate data. The failure of these instruments to deliver the expected insights was followed by a return to the earlier practice of treating the literal meanings of a person's statements as a valid proxy for behavioral data. This premise is often invalidated and, on occasion, leads to starkly counterintuitive conclusions.

The explanations offered for the many documented relations between an early experience and a psychological outcome assume that the events the subjects described actually occurred, not that a person said they occurred. No biologist would rely only on the reports of hunters for inferences about the ecology of a forest. Humans have been talking about the relations between traits and experiences, one the one hand, and later outcomes for millennia. If this evidence provided the foundation for profound conclusions, we should have a deeper understanding of human personality than we do.

The critical function of theory is to evaluate the validity of statements based on different evidence and select the one that should be awarded the greatest trust. Theory awards priority to the inference that the human use of fossil fuels is one reason why the Greenland glaciers are melting. Unfortunately, investigators who study brain–mind relations cannot agree on theoretical ideas powerful enough to sort inferences into categories that are more rather than less trustworthy. There is still considerable controversy surrounding the psychological meaning of activation of the fusiform area to pictures of faces. This issue is discussed in chapter 4.

The validity of cause–effect claims is also burdened by the habit of looking for relations between single causes and single outcomes. Thousands of papers describe the relation between one risk factor—say, growing up with a depressed parent or being a victim of bullying—and a single outcome, whether a teacher's rating of asocial behavior, the cortisol wakening response, heart rate, or the BOLD signal to a brain site. Inferences based on *patterns* of causes and outcome variables provide a sounder basis for theory, because most behaviors and brain profiles are the product of more than one cascade of events. Patterns of causes and outcome measures are needed to parse all the possible cascades into a number of distinct sequences.

The symptoms that lead to a diagnosis of autism, for example, can be the product of a very large number of distinct cascades involving different genes and gene expressions. The task is to discover each of these, one by one. It is likely that, at the end of this mission, clinicians and investigators will cast aside the term *autism*. (Few, if any, contemporary psychiatrists use the older diagnostic term *neurasthenia*.)

A person's social class during the childhood years is almost always an element in the patterns that predict many of the outcomes a majority of societies care about. When childhood social class is added to gender and ethnicity, the probability of pathology developing in youth who grew up with a depressed parent is increased considerably. A pattern that combines growing up in an economically disadvantaged family with being the victim of sexual abuse is a better predictor of maladaptive habits than either one of those conditions.

The use of covariance techniques to justify the awarding of causal influence to a single condition is questionable because investigators who rely on these statistics usually fail to meet the trio of requirements: linear relations among variables, the absence of outliers, and a priori specification of all expected outcomes. As a result, strange conclusions are often disseminated. One group of scientists relying on such a statistical manipulation concluded that the residents of Louisiana are the most satisfied Americans. Another group found that the probability of suicide was highest in nations with the largest number of psychiatrists. Biological phenomena reveal the danger of an unreflective reliance on covariance techniques. No biologist would use covariance to control for altitude, rainfall, and hours of sunshine in order to arrive at an estimate of the influence of genes on the heights of five genetic strains of a plant because they know that the covariates have nonlinear relations to the heights of each strain.

Investigators should consider replacing their current emphasis on single continuous variables with patterns of traits that define classes of persons. Instead of looking for a correlation between the scores on the neuroticism scale of the Big Five questionnaire and the risk for developing anorexia, it will prove more profitable to create categories that combine gender, class, ethnicity, language ability, and neuroticism score. We need more studies that allow authors to write, "Adolescent females from an advantaged family group who have vocabulary scores above the median and high values on the neuroticism scale of the Big Five are at the highest risk for an eating disorder." Chapter 5 documents the power of patterns.

The practice of borrowing predicates whose meanings and validities originated in psychological measures gathered on human subjects and applying them to brain patterns, or to animals, rounds out the constraints to be considered. Gyorgy Buzsaki (2016), a sophisticated student of the brain, questions the wisdom of attributing any psychological process to a neuronal ensemble. Most sentences containing a predicate that presumes a human as the noun possess a distinctive meaning and validity that does not apply to brain sites or animals. The meaning of the predicate *fears* in a sentence describing the emotion of a woman who avoids parties differs from the meaning of the same word in a sentence describing the increased BOLD signal to the amygdala of an adult looking at pictures of snakes and spiders.

Investigators who award animals a psychological quality that has a unique meaning in humans are guilty of an equally misleading permissiveness. The term *aggression* furnishes an example. Aggressive acts committed by humans assume an intention to harm another. A nursing infant who bites her mother's nipple has not committed an aggressive act, even though the mother felt pain. A cat that initially paws and subsequently bites the neck of a mouse did not intend to harm it. Lions bite the neck of gazelles because they are hungry. They hold no animosity toward the gazelle they killed.

One reason for these misattributions is that neuroscientists do not have a vocabulary large enough to describe the varied patterns of brain activation to an incentive. An unexpected picture of a snake typically excites the amygdala, hippocampus, and visual and prefrontal cortex. This pattern needs a biological name. Instead of inventing that name, investigators borrow the psychologist's concept of fear. When biologists discovered that methyl groups on cytosine bases adjacent to guanine in promoter regions could affect a gene's expression, they invented a new term to describe this fact.

A deeper understanding of the brain's contribution to mental and behavioral outcomes requires investigators to acknowledge these five constraints, which are rarely considered together in the design or interpretation of an experiment.

Every author imagines a prototypical reader sitting on a shoulder studying the prose being typed. My audience for this book was the collection of active scientists and students in the social sciences, psychiatry, or neuroscience. I learned a great deal in the writing of this book. The gratification would be enhanced if any idea in the chapters that follow changed a single mind.

2   The Power of the Context

Every event occurs in a setting in which a small number of reactions are highly probable and a large number improbable (Horner, Bisby, Wang, Bogus, & Burgess, 2016). The setting includes not only the physical and social features of the location, but also the procedure generating the evidence which influences the expectations of the subjects.

The early differentiation of the cells of the mammalian blastocyst, formed soon after fertilization, is an exquisite example of the power of context. The spatial position of each cell during the transition from 8 to 16 cells renders the cells facing the outside environment less contractile than those facing inward. The former become the placenta. The more contractile cells forming the inner mass will differentiate into the animal's organs and limbs (Maitre, Tuilier, Illukkumbura, Eismann, Niwayama, Nedelec, & Hiragi, 2016). Why a cell's spatial position determines its contractility remains a mystery.

Contextual Constraints on Brain Profiles

The laboratories that measure brain activity contain uncommon combinations of physical features and incentives that prime some brain sites and suppress others. The neurons primed by an expectation of physical harm are suppressed in individuals in a laboratory looking at pictures of snakes but are primed when the same person is hiking in a forest known to have dangerous snakes. On the other hand, the sites primed by the knowledge that strangers are evaluating one's performance are likely to be activated in individuals lying in a magnetic scanner being asked various questions.

Despite these possibilities, neuroscientists continue to speculate about the implications of the brain patterns they record as if the context has a minimal influence on their observations. This position is difficult to defend given the fact that the parahippocampal cortex binds objects and events to the context in which they appear (Aminoff, Kveraga, & Bar, 2013; Rath, Wurnig, Fischmeister, Klinger, Hollinger, Geibler, et al., 2016).

Adults lying supine and still in the narrow tube of a magnetic scanner in an unfamiliar room are in an unusual psychological and bodily state. The compromised sense of agency, awareness of being evaluated, confinement in a narrow space, and the demand to suppress all movement affect brain and psychological processes (Civile & Obhi, 2016; Hobson & Inzlicht, 2016). It is unlikely that the brain's reaction to a gray-scale male face with a fearful expression, devoid of a body and a background, would resemble the pattern generated, if it could be measured, when these same subjects saw a man with a fearful facial expression running out of an office building (Lee & Siegle, 2014).

There are many reasons for this claim. The most important is that the context, defined by a man running out of a building, triggered thoughts of potential danger that were absent while lying in the scanner. Settings, like switches in a circuit, select one sequence from a collection of alternatives. It is also relevant that the person walking by the building will be activating motor modules involved in locomotion and sites in sensory cortex responding to the noises of the traffic and the sights on the street and sidewalk. This activity necessarily affects the brain response to a fearful face. A less important reason is that the brain's hemodynamics in a supine posture differ from the values recorded when the same adults are in a sitting or standing position (Thibault, Lifshitz, & Raz, 2016; Spironelli, Busenello, & Angrilli, 2016).

The incentive and the examiner's instruction have a palpable effect on the brain profile (Balaban & Luria, 2016; Depue, Orr, Smolker, Naaz, & Banich, 2016). Adults who were told that a computer program composed a selection of music generated a brain response that differed from the reaction in subjects who believed the same piece of music was composed by a person (Schindler & Kissler, 2016; Schindler, Wegrzyn, Steppacher, Kissler, 2015;see also Fabbri, Stubbs, Cusack, & Culham, 2016; Kim & McCarthy, 2016). Many investigators would like to discover the brain circuits that are the foundation of decontextualized emotional concepts, such as fear, joy, or anger. This mission is likely to fail because the brain pattern to a threat, source of pleasure, or frustration depends on the setting in which the incentive occurred (Clark-Polner, Johnson, & Barrett, 2016). Although oxytocin often creates a brain state which produces a feeling humans interpret as relaxed, there are exceptions (Churchland & Winkielman, 2012). Men given oxytocin when they were in a socially stressful situation reported feeling tense and displayed increased blood flow to the cingulate cortex (Eckstein, Scheele, Weber, Stoffel-Wagner, Maier, & Hurlemann, 2014). The setting provides agents with the information they need to infer the correct emotional state or thoughts of individuals displaying certain facial expressions or postures. Earlier investigators had labeled these phenomena as products of the "demand characteristics of the situation" (Sharpe & Whelton, 2016).

The setting has equally significant effects on animals. The neuronal activity in the medial frontal cortex of rats performing a sequence of three, over-learned responses in a maze differed from the pattern recorded when the animals executed the same trio of behaviors in a chamber (Ma, Hyman, Durstewitz, Phillips, & Seamans, 2016). The behaviors of rats given an antagonist to the vasopressin receptor depended on whether the animals were in their familiar home cage or an unfamiliar setting (Bredewold, Smith, Dumais, & Veenema, 2014).

The place cells in a rat's hippocampus that fire when an animal in search of food is running out of an arm in a maze differ from those that are active when it is running into that arm (Korte & Schmitz, 2016). Graybiel (2008) reminds her colleagues that the sites that are active when an animal is learning a new behavior are not necessarily the sites that are activated after the behavior has become habitual.

The Collection of Events

The particular collection of incentives affects both psychological and brain profiles. Adult ratings of the unpleasantness of a word or the quality of a texture depend on the particular set of comparisons presented (Kamp, Potts, & Donchin, 2015; Heaps & Handel, 1999). Dutch students selecting the two most closely related words from a trio of unrelated nouns chose different pairs when the words in the triad varied (De Deyne, Navarro, Perfors, & Storms, 2016). Consider, as an example, the word most European adults would pair with the word *coffee*. If *coffee* appeared with *lion* and *box* most would choose *lion* because both are found in Africa. But if it appeared with *lion* and *pizza* more would select *pizza* because both are foods. If it occurred with *box* and *cat* a majority would pair it with *cat* because both begin with the same letter. If *coffee* appeared with *cat* and *night* a majority would pick *night* because both are dark. And if it appeared with *cat* and *kindness* most subjects would select *kindness* because both are associated with pleasure.

A face with a fearful expression evokes a large response from the amygdala when it appears with non-fearful faces. The amygdalar response is considerably smaller when the same fear face is part of a collection that contains scenes symbolic of fear (Schafer, Schienle, & Vaitl, 2005). Neutral video clips generate the largest event-related waveforms and the most activity in the corrugator muscle when presented with pleasant and unpleasant videos because they are the only non-emotional stimuli (Wiggert, Wilhelm, Reichenberger, & Blechert, 2015; Lee, Kang, Park, Kim, & An, 2008).

Infants displayed an increase in pupil diameter when they heard an infrequent 750 Hz tone in an oddball paradigm that contained many examples of a standard 500 Hz tone. However, they failed to display an increase in pupil diameter when the same 750 Hz tone was presented along with the more salient sounds of a crying infant and a phone ringing because it was now less deviant from the standard (Wetzel, Buttelmann, Schieler, & Widmann, 2016).

The reliance on a single collection of incentives limits the scientist's ability to generalize conclusions. Many investigators had concluded that the fusiform face area was especially tuned to respond to faces. However, when other investigators presented additional examples of frequently encountered events that contained meaningful details within a larger array they found that these, too, activated this site. For example, adults reading words, chess experts looking at arrays of pieces on a chessboard, and experienced radiologists examining X-rays display fusiform activation (Axelrod, 2016; Bilalic, 2016; Bilalic, Grottenthaler, Nagele, & Lindig, 2016).

Contextual Constraints on Behavior

The immediate setting modulates decisions, voice quality, facial expression, fluency, cooperation, emotional state, expression of an operant, working memory, magnitude of startle, perception, color preferences, the blocking phenomenon, and preferential attention to a novel versus a familiar stimulus (van Maanen, Forstmann, Keuken, Wagenmakers, & Heathcote, 2016; Shields & Rovee-Collier, 1992; Silva, Chein, & Steinberg, 2016; Gregory & Webster, 1996; Odegaard & Shams, 2016; Soussignan & Schall, 1996; Bartz, 2016; Kayal, Widen, & Russell, 2015; Rodger, Vizioli, Ouyang, & Caldera, 2015; Weidemann, Satkunarajah, & Lovibond, 2016; Sharif & Oppenheimer, 2016; Piantadosi, Kidd, & Aslin, 2014; Ramenzoni & Liszowski, 2016; Schacter & Singer, 1962; Kamin, 1969).

The meaning of a word or phrase typically depends on the other words in the sentence that supply a context (van Dam, van Dongen, Bekkering, & Rueschemeyer, 2012; Hoffman, Lambon, & Rogers, 2013). The phrase *The cat is on* has a different meaning in each of the following sentences: "The cat is on the floor of the morgue in the veterinarian's office," "The cat is on the roof of a moving car," and "The cat is on her side nursing her litter" (Putnam, 2012). Although there was no relation between the familiarity and meaningfulness of a metaphor when Italian students read the metaphor in its original literary context, these measures were positively related when the metaphor was read in isolation (Bambini, Resta, & Grimaldi, 2014).

The setting preferentially primes the networks that have a high probability of being activated by a particular word. Consider the term *oxygen*. A woman visiting a sick friend who is receiving oxygen will activate networks for hospitals, illness, and life. A student reading about the discovery of oxygen is likely to activate networks for laboratories, candles, and perhaps Lavoisier. A woman who was thinking about bells while walking by a church might activate the network for death if she remembered that John Donne was thinking of church bells ringing to signal someone's death when he wrote, "never send to know for whom the bell tolls, it tolls for thee."

Decision theorists hoping to discover rules governing the most rational choice in diverse settings have been frustrated because a decision to avoid or assume risk depends on the person, the context, and for bilingual adults the language used to pose the problem. The probabilities of an automobile accident because a driver ignored a red light at 3:00 a.m. on a deserted street and winning a national lottery are equally low, but many drivers who stop for the red light buy lottery tickets.

The presence of blue lights at a Japanese railway station reduced the incidence of suicide over a 13-year interval (Matsubayashi, Sawada, & Ueda, 2014). One reason may be that exposure to blue light reduces activity in anterior cingulate cortex during a state of uncertainty (Alkozei, Smith, & Killgore, 2016). Adults in a scanner trying to detect the occasions when a neutral or smiling face was repeated relied on variation in the eyebrows and facial shadows to solve the problem (Nestor, Plaut, &

Behrmann, 2016). They would not use eyebrows and facial shadows to detect the face of a friend at a large party (Passingham, Rowe, & Sakai, 2012). Perceptual decisions made in a scanner are characterized by longer response latencies and more errors compared with performance on the same task outside the scanner (van Maanen, Forstmann, Keuken, Wagenmakers, & Heathcote, 2016). Even the many demonstrations of the blocking effect, first introduced by Kamin (1969), are not replicated when small changes are made in the procedure (Maes, Boddez, Alfei, Kryptos, D'Hooge, De Houwer, & Beckers, 2016).

A detail as seemingly irrelevant as the size of the room affects the feature in the room that two-year-olds use in looking for a hidden object (Learmonth, Newcombe, & Huttenlocher, 2001). One-year-olds do not cry when their mother leaves them through a door in the home that she normally uses, but are more likely to cry if she leaves by a door rarely taken or by a door in an unfamiliar laboratory room.

Three-month-old infants can discriminate between the weights of heavy and light objects when tested in a dark room, but cannot do so in a lit room (Striano & Bushnell, 2005). Recordings of the utterances of one child, from his first word at nine months to two years, along with the speech to which he was exposed, revealed that the child was most likely to repeat a new word when an adult spoke that word in a unique context. The words diaper, poop, breakfast, door, and medicine are examples of words that the child heard in a distinctive setting (Roy, Frank, DeCamp, Miller, & Roy, 2015).

School-age children making judgments about the fairness of the distribution of resources favor equity when the recipients vary in competence, effort expended, or need, but prefer equality when these conditions are irrelevant (Sigelman & Waitzman,

1991). Children's play groups in villages in less developed societies often contain a large age range and some adults nearby. As a result, there are many occasions when an older child nurtures a younger one who is upset and few instances of fighting. The former are less and the latter more frequent in urban settings where play groups contain a restricted range of age and no adults.

The day of the week and the time of day were the best predictors of what a person was doing when a smartphone signal instructed a large sample of young adults to record their activity (Taquet, Quoidbach, de Montjoye, Desseilles, & Gross, 2016). The same is true for hyenas. Observations of spotted hyenas in an African national park over a 20-year interval revealed that the immediate setting, not the animal's family pedigree, accounted for most of the variance in the frequency of approaches to a lion that was near a food source and biting, lunging, or snapping at another hyena (Yoshida, Van Meter, & Holekamp, 2016).

Climate appears to affect the likelihood that a community will adopt a tonal language. More societies in the hot, humid climates of central Africa and southern China have tonal languages than do those in cold, dry regions. It is easier to adjust the vocal system to make the subtle changes necessary for tonal forms when the mouth is moist rather than dry (Lupyan & Dale, 2016).

The context has equally persuasive influences on animals. A monkey's performance on a simple task is enhanced when a familiar monkey is present. The behaviors of older monkeys whose amygdalae had been lesioned a few days after birth were dissimilar because the animals were raised and assessed in slightly different settings (Amaral & Adolphs, 2016). Whether one bonobo chimpanzee dominates another depends on whether they form a dyad or a third animal is present (Vervaecke, de Vries, & van

Elsacker, 1999). Primatologists believe that the distinctly different social behaviors of chimpanzees (*Pan troglodytes*) and their
close relative the bonobos are due partly to the fact that the
ecology of the bonobos has a richer food supply. The relaxed
burden on survival in the bonobo settings was accompanied
by the selection of a distinctive pattern of traits (Takuyama &
Furuichi, 2016). A species of coral reef fish living near Australia's
Heron Island provides a dramatic example of the power of the
social setting. The dominant female in the harem undergoes a
sex reversal when the single male dies (Robertson, 1972).

One reason for the modest effects of most intervention projects with children or youth who exhibit psychological problems is that the intervention usually occurs in a quiet room in
a school, Head Start center, or university laboratory. The child's
maladaptive behaviors, however, occur with peers or at home
(Dodge, 2011). Effective programs implemented by one group of
psychologists often fail when a different group of investigators
apply the same rituals with another sample because the contexts
have been altered. Slight changes in one aspect of a procedure
are an important cause of the many failures to replicate the
results of an original study (Savage, Becker, & Lipp, 2016). When
the contexts are very similar, the replication is more often successful (Van Bavel, Mende-Siedlecki, Brady, & Reinero, 2016).

Richard Shweder described a remarkable example of the
power of context in a talk at Harvard in 2000. Shweder and his
wife were living temporarily in the Indian temple town of Orissa
where he was doing field work. Because their dinner guests possessed different statuses he had to make sure that the food was
acceptable to all three by going to a local temple and gathering
food that others had placed there earlier. Anyone is allowed to eat
a food once a god has removed its essence. Some rice remained

in the bowl after the guests had left, and his wife diced chicken into the bowl and served it to Richard. Surprisingly, he could not suppress a feeling of disgust that prevented him from eating. Shweder's awareness of being in the dining room of a house in a temple town altered his emotion. He does not feel disgust when he eats chicken and rice in his Chicago home.

It would be instructive if scientists presented words, sentences, sounds, or pictures to subjects in different virtual environments. The results of such experiments would reveal whether brain patterns and behaviors vary as a function of the setting. Would the brain patterns and ratings of arousal to fearful, angry, disgusted, and happy faces in three different virtual contexts— say, a summer beach, a vacant city street at night, and an office with workers in cubicles—vary with the setting?

Range of Incentives

The range of stimuli presented can have significant consequences, especially when subjects are discriminating among similar events. Adults are able to detect the difference between lines 40 and 42 mm long when the lengths range from 35 to 45 mm. Surprisingly, they have difficulty detecting the same 2 mm difference when the range is extended to 20 to 60 mm (Namdar, Ganel, & Algon, 2016). The ability to detect small differences in the weights of pairs of objects honors the same principle. Simply extending the range of faces displaying pain reduced adult judgments of pain intensity (Gregoire, Coll, Tremblay, Prkachin, & Jackson, 2016). Most studies of infant cognition present only two test events—the familiarized stimulus and a novel one that alters a critical feature in the former. It would be informative if psychologists added a third stimulus that was a slight variation on the familiar and a fourth test event that was totally unrelated to the familiar one. Most infants look longest at slight variations on their past experience and least at stimuli that share no features with their knowledge (Kagan, Kearsely & Zelazo, 1978). Individuals acting in their usual settings typically have more than one choice when they have to decide whether to cooperate with another. As a result they do not always behave as they do in games like Prisoner's Dilemma (Stewart, Parsons & Plotkin, 2016).

Anxious patients prompted at irregular times during the day to report the emotion they were experiencing at that moment were less differentiating than healthy adults in the terms used to describe an unpleasant feeling (Kashdan & Farmer, 2014). One explanation is that adults with social anxiety disorder experience a broader range of feelings during most months than minimally anxious persons.

Children are less accepting of slight deviations in the ways people eat, dress, or talk than adults because of their restricted exposure to adult behaviors. The extreme reactions some autistic children show to slight deviations from the familiar may reflect their restricted range of experience (Trueblood, Brown, Heathcote, & Bisemeyer, 2013). Replies to questions about a child's personality given by parents who have raised three children differ from those given by parents of one child because the former have dealt with a larger range of moods, demands, and behaviors.

I suspect that the limited exposure to serious loss, trauma, threat, or frustration is one reason for the large number of contemporary adolescents and young adults from comfortable, middle-class families complaining of anxiety or depression. Twenty-year-olds who have enjoyed comfortable circumstances most of their lives rely on a relatively narrow range of feelings when they reflect on a hostile comment by a peer or an upcoming exam. This restricted range of emotions tempts them to exaggerate the seriousness of a small deviation from their normally pleasant feeling tone. By contrast, young adults who have suffered both harsh and pleasant events on many occasions are less likely to interpret the feeling that follows a rude remark or task failure as implying a state that deserves attention. Hispanic and black youth from Chicago neighborhoods who experienced frequent violence reported less anxiety than youths of the same ethnicity who had been exposed to minimal violence (Kennedy & Ceballo, 2016).

Before potable water and antibiotics an infectious disease often killed a large proportion of the residents of a community. Youths who lost a parent to cholera are unlikely to be overly concerned with a snub, a criticism, or a frustration. A woman who spent her childhood and adolescence on one of Britain's Council Estates for working class residents in the 1980s wrote, "The more you shrink your own world, the more likely you are to be frightened by the unexpected" (Hanley, 2016, p. 45).

The range of experiences shapes judgments about the morality of an individual or an action. Americans living in small towns in less densely populated regions hold more conservative views on parental responsibilities, teenage pregnancies, illegal immigrants, gay marriage, and abortion than adults in large cities who are exposed to a broad range of violations of traditional moral standards. Many members of the Ku Klux Klan in the 1920s lived in towns in the Midwest that had few blacks, Eastern European Jews, or supporters of the communist ideology of the Soviet Union (Boehm & Corey, 2015).

Television, laptops, and iPhones expose millions of viewers to scenes or descriptions of explicit sexuality, the aftermath of earthquakes and hurricanes, the rubble of Syrian and Iraqi cities, the terrible conditions of refugees, the massacres in select cities, corpses in buses charred by suicide bombers, gang rapes of women in college dormitories, Ponzi schemes that robbed victims of their life savings, an executive of an important institution requesting oral sex from a chamber maid, and employees of investment firms lying to clients. The awareness of these events mutes worry over a house fire in the neighborhood, a stabbing outside a bar, the prevalence of pornography, or women masturbating with a sex toy, even though these violations of the traditional moral standards existing a century earlier would have generated guilt in the agent or anger toward the perpetrator.

The more lenient parental punishments of young children for violations of norms on cleanliness and bodily products since the 1950s probably contributed to the currently permissive posture toward those who fail to conform to local standards. Nineteenth-century middle-class American mothers imposed harsh punishments on toddlers who played with their feces or vomit and were likely to add, "That's disgusting." This experience established an association between violation of a moral standard and the neural network for the concept of disgust. The more permissive socialization practices of contemporary parents may have weakened this link. Most Americans who learn about genital mutilation, beheading of hostages, the sale of children for money, or the trafficking of young women for prostitution acknowledge that these practices are cruel, unfortunate, sad, or unjust, but are less likely than earlier generations to call them disgusting.

Contexts Select Symptoms

Each person's biology and childhood history create different kinds of vulnerabilities to varied psychological states. Some of these states make it difficult for a youth or adult to honor their society's expectations or demands. But the particular symptoms vulnerable children or adults acquire are determined, in many instances, by their life circumstances at the time. This suggestion means that the diagnostic category clinicians assign to patients has an important origin in the contexts the patient encounters regularly. There would be far fewer cases of substance abuse disorder in communities without easy access to alcohol, cocaine, or opioids. The prevalence of gambling disorder or erotomania would be small if there were no websites allowing gambling or showing pornographic films. If children did not have to attend school there would be fewer cases of ADHD. The frequency of binge drinking in the United States in 2015 was highest in states with low population densities and cold winters, such as Alaska, Montana, the Dakotas, and New Hampshire, and less common in warm southern states with denser populations.

The results of a 30-year longitudinal study of three generations that began with a sample of depressed and healthy adults is relevant. The members of the third generation who had a mental illness and, in addition, a depressed grandparent and parent displayed a variety of symptoms. Although some were depressed, others had an anxiety or substance abuse disorder (Weissman, Berry, Warner, Gameroff, Skipper, Talati, Pilowsky & Wickamaratne, 2016). A study of more than 800,000 Danes revealed that when both a parent and an adolescent offspring had a psychiatric illness, their diagnoses were frequently dissimilar because each had to cope with different circumstances (Dean, Stevens & Mortensen, 2010).

Anorexia in the United States and Europe is most common among white females from middle- or upper-middle class families who were socialized to accomplish something of importance and to maintain control of their lives (Haworth-Hoeppner, 2017; Goodman, Heshmati, & Koupil, 2014). Because the feeling that follows a perception of loss of control is threatening, it motivates an attempt to reassure the self that it has regained some measure of control. The ability to restrain the amount of food eaten is one way to meet this need.

Consider a young woman with a vulnerability to uncertainty who grew up in an upper-middle class family in a small town. The decision to attend a large university in a major city would render her susceptible to a feeling of lost control over the day's events. As a result, she might decide to control her eating as a way to assure herself that she retains some control. If this habit continues for many months she might develop the symptoms of anorexia. On the other hand, if the same woman did not leave her home and instead developed a romantic relationship with a man who exploited and eventually betrayed her, she might experience guilt over her failure to detect the man's character and, as a result, develop a depression rather than anorexia.

The adults born with a temperamental susceptibility to chronic tension could acquire a mood of anger or guilt depending on how their past history and current circumstances shaped the interpretation they imposed on a tension with an ambiguous origin.

The anxiety or depression reported by adolescents who are targets of malicious gossip from members of their social network has been potentiated by the availability of the Internet. The high anxiety among high school students desiring admission to prestigious colleges is a relatively recent phenomenon brought on by the increased numbers of high school seniors applying to a small number of schools. This level of worry was far less common 50 years ago.

The anger at those holding elite positions in politics, science, the media, or business felt by a proportion of Americans who did not graduate college is due, partly, to the tendency to turn against those who are believed to be a source of guilt or shame. The higher incomes and privileged status enjoyed by a large proportion of college graduates with technical skills remind those with only a high school diploma and a modest income of their vocational failure in a society that equates virtue with wealth and education. Hence, they blame the former for their unhappy state. Novelists often exploit this dynamic. The youth Amir in *The Kite Runner* (by Khaled Hosseini) turns against his friend Hassan because he is the source of Amir's guilt that began when he failed to save his friend from a vicious attack by a gang of bullies.

Chronic guilt can lead to a serious depression if the person cannot find an activity that allows some form of penance. Those who live in settings that make it easier to find a mission that assures them of their moral virtue—Mahatma Gandhi is an example—are protected from serious depression. These examples point to the influence of contexts, which are often limited to a given culture during a particular historical era, on the patterns of emotions and habits that clinicians diagnose as a mental illness.

Study of the biological properties and childhood experiences that contribute to an outcome should be balanced with detailed examination of the contexts that youth and adults confront each day. The failure to recognize that a majority of individuals assigned to a psychiatric category could have been given a different diagnosis had their current conditions been different is hampering discovery of the major vulnerabilities. The search for the genes that contribute to a mental illness category in the Diagnostic and Statistical Manual of Mental Disorders (DSM-5) should be replaced with a search for the genes that contribute to the many vulnerabilities. Some biological signs of these vulnerabilities, called endophenotpyes, are level of activity in the hypothalamic pituitary axis, the balance between sympathetic and parasympathetic activity, EEG profiles, wave five in the brain stem auditory evoked potential, and level of corrugator muscle tension in uncertain settings (Kagan & Snidman, 2004).

Neighborhoods, Regions, and Nations

Neighborhoods vary in the temptations and challenges their residents encounter. The fights, murders, and affronts to maleness that are common in select cities invite violence in young men whose vocational futures are uncertain (Ellis, 2016). Such men find it difficult to withdraw from a challenge to fight because the anticipated shame that would follow a failure to honor the ethical demand to be tough is regarded as far more distressing than the pain of a fight. The reason why the homicide rate is higher in Chicago than in New York is that the psychological boundaries between poor and wealthy neighborhoods are less permeable in Chicago (Venkatesh, 2013).

The geographic region within a nation affects a variety of outcomes. The probability of receiving a diagnosis of ADHD varies significantly across the 50 American states, with rates as high as 1 in 7 in North Carolina and Alabama but only 1 in 17 in Nevada and California (Centers for Disease Control and Prevention,

2007). The probability that an adult with an income in the top fifth of the distribution grew up in a family whose income was in the bottom fifth was highest in San Francisco, Seattle, and New York and lowest in Cleveland, Detroit, and Atlanta (Leonhardt, 2013).

Older South Koreans living in a poor, rural region are at a high risk for suicide because many of their sons and daughters have left them to work in a city (Chan, Caine, You, & Yip, 2015). Older adults who live alone in rural regions of western Europe have lower suicide rates because they enjoy more adequate social support. Older adults in wealthy nations report that they are happier than younger ones. In poor nations, however, the younger adults report being happier (Swift, Vauclair, Abrams, Bratt, Marques, & Lima, 2014).

The cultural setting even influences the evaluation of the intelligence of someone displaying a smile. Europeans judge such faces as intelligent but East Asians do not (Krys, Melanie-Vauclair, Capaldi, Lun, Bond, Dominque-Espinosa et al., 2016). Adolescents from isolated, island communities in New Guinea and Mozambique found it difficult to pick out the one face from sets of six faces that was expressing an emotion synonymous with the English words fear, sad, disgust, angry, or happy (Crivelli, Jarillo, Russell, & Fernandez-Dols, 2016). American and European youths find the same task easy.

The setting assumes special significance in Japanese society. A person in a public place is expected to adopt the posture of *tatemae*, which calls for politeness and formality, even with a spouse, child, or old friend. The informal, candid posture of *honne* is appropriate in the home. The Japanese award more power to the workplace setting than do Americans. No American court would fine the company of an employee who committed suicide because working overtime for many weeks at the request of his employer created a deep depression. But that is exactly what a Japanese superior court did in 2000 (Kitanaka, 2012).

An isolated tribe in New Guinea provides a persuasive example of the influence of a culture on the interpretation of behavior (Herdt, 1994). The members of this small community believe that all boys are born sterile. In order to acquire the seed necessary to father children, the preadolescent boys perform fellatio on the older, unmarried males for about six or seven years. No boy views this behavior as a sign of homosexuality or gender identity confusion.

Historical Changes in Contexts

The cyclical changes in temperature and rainfall across various regions have had dramatic consequences on the locations of the major civilizations. Had the glaciers not receded from northern Europe by 10 to 15,000 years ago, the domestication of barley, wheat, sheep, and goats in the Middle East would not have occurred and the famous civilizations of that region would not have been established.

The contexts that characterize a historical era within a society have profound effects on beliefs, values, behaviors, and worries. Luther's sixteenth-century rebellion against the Catholic Church was a watershed moment because it implied that no person or institution, no matter how powerful, was protected from challenge. It is not a coincidence that the natural sciences exploded during the next two centuries. The devastation, death, and unrest wrought by the Thirty Years War, which turned seventeenth-century Europeans against the occult declarations of religious leaders, made the public more receptive to the empirical discoveries of Galileo, Harvey, and Newton.

The ideas spawned by scientific discoveries and explanations were requisites for John Locke's thesis that each person begins life with few biases. It is a short leap from this idea to Thomas Jefferson's declaration that all men are created equal and entitled to liberty and the pursuit of whatever they decide will bring them happiness. The public was less pleased, however, when twentieth-century physicists and biologists announced that all life was an accident with no ulterior purpose other than to beget the next generation. This pessimistic message, when added to the horrors of two world wars and the irrational decisions by the leaders that brought on those wars, generated a skeptical posture toward any philosophical position defending a particular moral belief. In less than 500 years, historical events had replaced Luther's announcement that each person must seek salvation by good works with the dispiriting idea that all life goals and moral imperatives were simply human inventions that change with time and place.

The premises held by most sixteenth-century Europeans have been replaced in this century with a new collection among those living in economically developed democracies. The new ideology awards priority to the interests of the young over those of the old; insists that all persons are entitled to equal dignity independent of their sex, ethnicity, religion, or values; holds a prejudicial attitude toward many in positions of authority; has faith in the power of science and technology to solve all problems; is willing to believe that human existence has no special purpose or meaning; regards placing self's interests above the needs of others as a rational life strategy; and assumes happiness is a right rather than a matter of good luck.

When we add to these ideas the increasing inequalities in income and education, global warming, a world population approaching 8 billion with more than 80 percent of humans living in cities, increases in non-biodegradable garbage, pollution of air and water, and an information network that informs billions of individuals about an incident in a distant place, it is obvious that the current generation confronts a unique historical context that is marked by anonymity, a reduction in the occasions for shame, a reluctance to award any person a privileged moral authority, and belief in the wisdom of seizing an available pleasure now rather than wait for a better pleasure later (Bruckner, 2010; Twenge, Campbell, & Carter, 2014; Zijlema, Klijs, Stolk, & Rosmalen, 2015).

Current conditions in a large number of societies have led to a substantial rise in the number of adults who feel expendable. Arthur Miller captured this feeling of diluted potency when he had Willy Loman, the hapless husband and father in *Death of a Salesman,* complain, "I'm not noticed." Intellectual talents that were adaptive 150,000 years ago allowed our species to invent things that, over time, altered settings in ways that now compromise the psychic mood of millions of adults.

The changes in life style wrought by history have significantly influenced the popular forms of therapy for mental illnesses. During the nineteenth century, when "mental illness" usually meant a psychosis, material cures that altered the body were the most popular. Freud's ideas ascended during the first half of the last century as increasing numbers of Americans left small towns with agricultural economies for cities where the restraints on impulse that had been adaptive in their childhood settings were no longer appropriate. Freud's writings implied that those who worried excessively or lived with intrusive feelings of guilt were mentally ill. Psychoanalytic rituals promised to remove these inhibitions and allow clients to yield to temptations with minimal anxiety or guilt.

These rituals had lost their novelty by the end of the last century. More important, the uncertainties generated by the Cold War, nuclear bombs, the large-scale entry of mothers into the work force, the rise in the divorce rate, violent gangs, and life alone in large cities had generated bouts of depression that seemed to originate in life conditions rather than repressed sex or anger. The rituals of cognitive behavioral therapy seemed more appropriate for these symptoms. The increased popularity of the rituals of mindfulness therapy, a derivative of Buddhist philosophy, appears to be a response to an accelerated pace of life pervaded with intense competition. It is impossible to predict the type of therapy that will attract patients at the end of this century because we do not know what history's muse will arrange.

The emphasis on equality, especially in Europe and North America, was accompanied by a reduction in the symbolic significance of the rituals that separated youths from adults, educated from less educated, single from married, married women from mothers, and followers from leaders. The diluted emotion attached to these rituals created a subtle but annoying uncertainty about the responsibilities of those who have never participated in a high school or college commencement, a formal wedding in a religious setting, a party celebrating the birth of an infant, or a ceremony when someone assumed a position of authority. Youths understood that they were free to act as they wished and to regard themselves as worthy as anyone in their community. But some remained unsure of what they were supposed to do with these gifts. Rituals make it easier to accept the responsibilities attached to a role and, in so doing, dilute the tension that trails the temptation to surrender to the premise of "anything goes."

Uncertainty pierces consciousness when there is ambiguity over whom you can dominate and to whom you ought to be subordinate. A related state occurs in baboons and macaque monkeys. Baboons in troops with a stable dominance hierarchy show fewer signs of stress than animals in troops with unstable ranks. Rhesus macaques belonging to stable groups usually flee screaming when attacked by a dominant animal. Victims in less stable groups, which often collapse, attack the animal that bit them (Beisner, Jin, Fushing, & Mccowan, 2015). Status hierarchies in Japan are far more stable than they are in the United States, and citizen attacks on public buildings are rare in Japan.

Historical changes affect the functions of institutions. The parish church in seventeenth-century Europe served as arsenal, school, storehouse, fire station, fortress, library, source of economic aid, and playground (Kaplan, 2007). The loss of secure, well-paying, blue-collar jobs in the manufacturing sector of the American economy over the past 40 years made colleges and universities more important because all youth had to learn the technical skills required by the new economy.

Science before 1940 consisted primarily of single investigators, aided perhaps by one or two junior assistants, working in an academic setting. The natural sciences in 2016 are a collective enterprise in which large numbers of junior and senior investigators collaborate in a university, commercial enterprise, or government agency. The latter two contexts have become more prevalent as the number of PhDs in the natural sciences became larger than the number of openings for faculty positions. As a result, younger scientists began to award greater priority to securing a tenured professorship than to making an important discovery. Because publishing many papers in the small number of high-impact journals was regarded as a path to the prized goal, a large number of junior investigators designed experiments that had a high probability of yielding a result that would be accepted by one of these journals (Fochler, Felt, & Muller, 2016).

The experiments performed on the Large Hadron Collider required the skills of such a large number of scientists it was not clear who was responsible for judging whether a result ought to be published. In many cases, the director of the laboratory, who had not performed the experiments, made the decision. Compare the present situation with an earlier era. Percy Bridgman, a 1946 Nobel laureate in physics who worked alone, believed that the investigator who gathered the data bore the responsibility of deciding whether an observation was valid (Holton, 2002). An essay in the journal *Nature* for March 10, 2016, advising scientists on ways to recruit the best collection of postdoctoral fellows and senior investigators, reveals the impossibility of honoring Bridgman's principle (Woolston, 2016). More serious is the increased number of published papers that rely on fraudulent data and ethically questionable practices designed to inflate an investigator's citations (Biagioli, 2016). Bridgman would weep if he knew what history's muse had done to his beloved institution.

History also affects our receptivity to ideas about human nature. Freud's notions were most attractive to British and American middle-class adults who had been socialized to adhere to the Protestant values on inhibition of sexual and aggressive feelings and actions. Bowlby (1950) invented the concept of attachment at a time when it was unusual for an infant to be cared for by someone other than the biological mother. Surrogate care is common in 2016 and infants placed in good-quality day care do not suffer from the dangers Bowlby predicted (Kagan, Kearsley, & Zelazo, 1978; Booth-LaForce & Roisman, 2014). These results and evidence on the consequences of forms of infant caretaking in African and Indonesian societies account for the decreasing popularity of the concepts of secure and insecure infant attachments (Otto & Keller, 2014).

The recent spate of research on the failure to regulate asocial behaviors furnishes another example of history's contribution to the attractiveness of a psychological concept. Before the First World War, many middle-class American and European parents practiced a relatively severe socialization of sexual and aggressive behaviors in children. Freud, who argued that a strict regimen generated guilt and anxiety, suggested that parents should allow children more freedom of expression. Parents, supported by the writings of popular authors and the media, took his advice. Because American youth in 2015 committed more murders, used more opioids and amphetamines, and engaged in more frequent oral and anal sex than adolescents of the first half of the last century, the regulation of impulsive behaviors has become more urgent (Lefkowitz, Vasilenko, & Leavitt, 2016; Casey & Caudle, 2013).

The rash of violence across the world has tempted some scientists to decontextualize the concept of aggression by ignoring the form of the behavior (whether gossip, rejection, dishonesty, stealing, hitting, biting, killing, sexual attack, or arson), the context (home, school, bar, or auditorium), the target (friend, stranger, or family member), and the agent (youth, adult, criminal, rat, mouse, monkey, fish, or fruit fly). Despite the extraordinary variation in actions, settings, targets, and agents one group of investigators saw no problem titling their review of diverse studies "Genetics of Aggressive Behavior: An Overview" (Veroude, Zhang-James, Fernandez-Castillo, Bakker, & Cormand, 2016).

The assumption that an inability to regulate impulses is a primary basis for violent actions by adolescents ignores two facts. First, a majority of aggressive youth regulate their behaviors in many settings. They keep secrets, plan attacks on a rival gang, and inhibit hostile acts toward members of their in-group. Social scientists are reluctant to acknowledge that many youths who are able to inhibit their violent behaviors do not choose to do so because the actions affirm a feeling of agency, prove their courage, or are necessary to maintain membership in a supportive peer group.

The Context and Economics

The weights that economists assign to each of the multiple factors in an economy are altered in response to changes in that society. Adam Smith's premise that the best society was one in which each person was maximally free to pursue their interests with minimal outside restraints was appropriate in eighteenth-century England. The small merchants in ethnically homogeneous cities and towns wanted the respect of the members of their community and, therefore, avoided a level of greed that would provoke criticism. Twenty-first-century CEOs of large national or global firms are less likely to feel shame when citizens or the media criticize their pricing practices.

The emergence of the discipline of economics, a century later, occurred at a time when physicists and mathematicians enjoyed the highest respect in the academy. As a result, the new members of this nascent field focused on ideas that could be expressed in mathematical equations in the hope that they would be treated with a similar level of respect. Their mission was made easier by the fact that they could assign numbers to the major variables of money supply, income, gross domestic product, employment rate, and inflation. The decision by many governments after World War II to collect statistical information on their economies was an important impetus for the rise of economics. The sudden availability of large corpora of data motivated mathematically talented social scientists to invent equations that might explain the evidence.

Although contemporary economists acknowledge that their formal mathematical models make assumptions about human decisions and behaviors that are known to be incorrect, and often fail to make correct predictions, they defend the reliance on those models by noting that they do predict some phenomena better than chance. However, the claim by some economists that a couple's decision to have a child is no different from the decision to purchase a new car ignores the fact that humans are motivated by more than material gain. Economists who think it is appropriate to compare the satisfaction generated by raising a child with the feeling that accompanies receipt of a large check assume that satisfaction is a single psychological state. It is not. A woman nursing her newborn infant, an athlete who has just won a gold medal at an Olympics, and a merchant who has just landed a lucrative contract represent three very distinct psychological states.

The history of economics is a narrative of the sequential replacement of one set of weights in mathematical models with another in order to accommodate to the new contexts that history created. These include new technologies, wars, national catastrophes, immigration, laws, and demographic changes.

The evolution of these models can be likened to the changes in a 250-year-old colonial house, which require removal of some rooms and the addition of new rooms in novel architectural styles. Economists are fond of a graph illustrating the rise in income and material comforts over the past 300 years, especially in capitalist economies. There is a positive correlation, in many societies, among six conditions: a participatory democracy, an uncorrupted judiciary, respect for the law, a free press, free public education, and economic growth. Most economists want to persuade the public that the last factor is the principal determinant of the other five. It is easy to argue, however, that the combination of the first five is responsible for the last.

I noted earlier that the art critic Arthur Danto (2009) recognized the influence of the historical context on the judgment of select objects as artistic products. In this era, but not a century earlier, a symmetrical arrangement of old tires is treated as a work of art in a museum, but not at a gas station. A broken violin in a glass case lying on an attic floor does not evoke an aesthetic feeling. But I had a profound aesthetic experience years ago when I saw a broken violin mounted on the wall of a Danish art museum. The ways in which the context of a historical era impose limitations on actions, beliefs, and feelings in a culture can be likened to the the restricted movements of cows enclosed in a corral of a particular size and shape.

The Defeat of the Gestalt Theorists

The founders of psychology in late-nineteenth-century Germany adopted a physicist's frame of mind as they searched for general laws governing sensation, perception, and memory that would transcend the settings in which the observations were made. Most American psychologists followed the European bias. Neither John Watson, Clark Hull, Neal Miller, Kenneth Spence, nor B. F. Skinner paid much attention to the context in which animals—usually white rats—ran through mazes, struck levers, or poked their snout into an opening in order to obtain a piece of food or a sip of water. Clark Hull's (1943) hope of being psychology's Isaac Newton is apparent in his equation $E = H \times D$. This lean formula, intended to apply to diverse species in varied contexts, stated that the strength of the excitatory potential (E) necessary for the expression of a behavior was a multiplicative function of the strength of the habit (H) and the intensity of the drive for the reward (D) given to the animal when the correct response was made. Hull's vaulting ambition remains popular. One respected team of neuroscientists invented an equally lean equation in 2016 that posited a nonspecific neural force, labeled "general arousal," that was a function of only two variables (Calderon, Kilinc, Maritan, Banaver, & Pfaff, 2016).

A small number of psychologists friendly to Gestalt ideas—Solomon Asch and Kurt Lewin were two members of this group—wrote about the power of the setting while the behaviorists were consolidating their approach (Wagemans, Elder, Kubovy, Palmer, Peterson, Singh, & von der Heydt, 2012). The perceived lightness of a stimulus, the length of a line, and the color of a surface were influenced by the lightness, length, or color of the surrounding regions, lines, or colors. Unfortunately, the message the Gestalt theorists intended was drowned out by the more popular concepts of the behaviorists and the Freudians, who typically ignored the context in which animals or humans behaved.

The evidence implicating the influence of the context is too persuasive to ignore. The settings in laboratories, cultures, and historical eras, added to the constraints imposed by a person's genes, early family experiences, and social class, select one outcome from an envelope of alternatives. That is why the context has to be part of every conclusion. Many neuroscientists and psychologists studying brain–mind relations are reluctant to take this suggestion seriously. These investigators continue to write sentences such as "The amygdala mediates fear," "The nucleus accumbens mediates reward," "The intraparietal sulcus mediates number," or "The hippocampus registers locations." These contextually naked statements contain no information on the agent, the setting, the procedure that generated the evidence, or the particular form taken by the fear, reward, number sense, or location. It is time to replace these ambiguous conclusions with full sentences.

3 Expectedness

The brains of awake animals and humans are continually anticipating the event that is most likely to occur in the next moment and priming the brain sites that normally respond to that event. Neurons in the occipital cortex of six-month-old infants who had learned that an object appeared after a particular sound were activated by the sound, even though the visual event did not occur (Emberson, Richards, & Aslin, 2015). The right occipital gyrus and fusiform area are primed in subjects who expect to see a face, as are neurons in the motor cortex of adults who expect to hear speech emanating from a static face (Swaminathan, MacSweeney, Boyles, Waters, Watkins, & Mottonen, 2013).

Rats trained to expect sucrose show increased activity in the gustatory cortex to a cue signaling the possibility of a sweet taste (Gardner & Fontanini, 2014). Rats expecting a painful stimulus display activity in the anterior cingulate (Wang, Zhang, Chang, Woodward, Baccala, & Luo, 2008). Rabbits display three distinct brain patterns in dorsal hippocampus and frontal cortex when the expected event is replaced by either an unfamiliar environment, object, or live animal (Fontani, Farabollini, & Carli, 1984).

It is easy to teach animals, as well as humans, to expect an improbable event and to respond appropriately. Infants required only 10 trials to learn to direct their gaze at a location that was incongruent with the direction of a hand's motion (Daum, Wronski, Harms, & Gredeback, 2016). Not surprisingly, species vary in their biological preparedness for and likely response to particular events. Human infants, for example, attend longer to melodies with consonant compared with dissonant chords (Zentner & Kagan, 1996).

An expectation of pain, a difficult task, an unpleasant picture, an air puff to the face, the sound of hands clapping, a metaphorical sentence, a caress, cocaine, an exemplar of a semantic category, or the benefit of a medicine each affects brain profiles as well as the speed and accuracy of perceptions (Mitchell, 2015; Timm, Schonwiesner, Schroger, & San Miguel, 2016; Mayer, Schwiedrzik, Wibral, Singer, & Melloni, 2016; Zanto, Clapp, Rubens, Karlsson, & Gazzaley, 2016; Sinke, Forkmann, Schmidt, Wiech, & Bingel, 2016; Cox, Meyers, & Sinha, 2004; Labrenz, Icenhour, Schlamann, Forsting, Bingel, & Elsenbruch, 2016; Lin, Hsieh, Yeh, Lee, & Niddam, 2013; Rommers, Dijkstra, & Bastiaansen, 2013; Ebisch, Ferri, & Gallese, 2014; Kufahl, Li, Risinger, Rainey, Piacentine, Wu, et al., 2008; Perera, George, Grammer, Janicak, Pascual-Leone, & Wirecki, 2016; Nordenskjold, Martensson, Pettersson, Heintz, & Landen, 2016; Willems, Frank, Nijhof, Hagoort, & van den Bosch, 2016; Schwarz, Pfister, & Buchel, 2016; Rhudy, Williams, McCabe, Rambo, & Russell, 2006; Fonteyne, Vervliet, Hermans, Baeyens, & Vansteenwegen, 2009; Hsieh, Stone-Elander, & Ingvar, 1999; Meyerhoff & Rohan, 2016; Sherman, Kanai, Seth, & VanRullen, 2016; Pecina, Bohnert, Sikora, Avery, Langenecker, Mickey, et al., 2015; Faasse, Martin, Grey, Gamble, & Petrie, 2015; Perri,

Berchicci, Lucci, Cimmino, Bello, & Di Russo, 2014; Bueti & Macaluso, 2010).

Adults expecting a large monetary reward after pressing a button secreted dopamine and executed the response with greater vigor (Rigoli, Chew, Dayan, & Dolan, 2016). The anticipation of a pleasant experience may create a more salient feeling in adolescents than in children or older adults because of the large increase in dopamine secretion at puberty (McCutcheon, Conrad, Carr, Ford, McGehee, & Marinelli, 2012). This phenomenon helps to explain youths' frequent seeking of new experiences.

A person who picks up a small metal ball and a large wooden ball with identical masses perceives the latter as heavier because she expects large objects to weigh more than small ones (Buckingham, Goodale, White, & Westwood, 2016). Observers watching a man holding a small ball move his arm upward as if to throw the ball in the air expect the object to rise. About one-third of college students were certain they saw the ball rise and then vanish, even though the man never released the ball (Kuhn & Rensink, 2016). Young children with closed eyes were told to detect where on their body an adult was going to touch them. Because they expected to be touched in only one place, they failed to detect the times when the adult touched them in two places. However, they had no trouble detecting both locations when the adult informed them ahead of time that she might touch them in two places (Nolan & Kagan, 1978). Many answers that an examiner regards as an error are reasonable replies from children or adults who expected a different question.

English speakers reading words with five or more letters anticipate an abstract rather than a concrete word because most abstract terms are longer than concrete ones (Reilly, Westbury,

Kean, & Peelle, 2012). Thomas Albright (2015) provided an interesting example of the role of expectation on perception. A bilingual listener who anticipates hearing a sentence spoken in French perceives, " Pas de lieu Rhone que nous." The same adult expecting an English speaker hears, "Paddle your own canoe."

The members of a society speaking the same language gradually acquire similar associations between successive sentence sequences that occur with modest to high transition probabilities. Hence, listeners and readers share similar expectations regarding the small envelope of sentences that are most likely to follow a particular sentence. When the expectations refer to invisible events, such as a person's mental state or a causal condition, they are called inferences. Judgments of the semantic coherence of a sequence of sentences are based on these expectations. Adults who have grown up in a society in which children learned different languages and encountered divergent experiences are likely to hold dissimilar judgments of the coherence of certain narratives. As the level of diversity increases, there is probably a tipping point at which segments of the population accept as coherent distinctively different arguments about the same phenomenon.

We expect a tomato to be red and clover to be green. A picture of a tomato and clover generate different neuronal profiles when both objects have a surface hue that is midway between red and green. Moreover, adults perceive this color to be redder than it actually is on a tomato but greener that it is on clover (Vandenbroucke, Fahrenfort, Meuwese, Scholte, & Lamme, 2016). These facts point to the difficulty of separating the brain's response to the event in the perceptual field from its response to the expected event. This evidence implies that block designs, which present different classes of events in distinct sets of trials, might provide evidence that differed from designs in which stimuli from different categories are presented in a random order (Miller, Hermes, Witthoft, Rao, & Ojemann, 2015; Gibbons, Schnuerch, & Stahl, 2016).

The Brain and the Unexpected

Unexpected events activate many brain sites, but especially the amygdala, hippocampus, prefrontal cortex, ventral tegmental area, and locus ceruleus. The difference in the oscillation frequencies evoked by the event anticipated and the one that occurs may be a critical cause of these activations (Ortuno, Grieve, Cao, Cudeiro, & Rivadulla, 2014; El Karoul, King, Sitt, Meyniel, Van Gaal, Hasboun, et al., 2015; Durschmid, Zaehle, Hinrichs, Heinze, Voges, Garrido, et al., 2016; Baumann, Borra, Bower, Cullen, Habas, Ivry et al., 2015; Cloutier, Gabrieli, O'Young, & Ambady, 2011; Brandt, Sommer, Krach, Bedenbender, Kircher, Paulus & Jansen, 2013).

The ventral tegmental area and substantia nigra, which secrete dopamine, and the locus ceruleus which secretes norepinephrine, send projections to the hippocampus that facilitate the establishment of firmer memories for unexpected events. The locus ceruleus of mice searching for the location of food in an enclosure became active when the animal encountered an unexpected change in the texture of the floor (Takeuchi, Duszkiewicz, Sonneborn, Spooner, Yamasaki, Watanabe, et al., 2016.

The influential Rescorla-Wagner model of conditioning is based on the power of the unexpected to recruit attention to the conditioned or unconditioned stimulus, and, as a result, enhance the probability of establishing an association between them (Rescorla & Wagner, 1972). Many events that function as rewards are unexpected surprises that recruit attention to them. That is why monkeys with a lesioned amygdala are impaired in learning a 2-choice, reversal task with varying rewards (Costa, Dal Monte, Lucas, Murray, & Averbeck, 2016).

The unexpected onset or offset of an event, whether pleasant or aversive, as well as an unexpected change in the amount or timing of a reward, are often followed by increases in dopamine, acetylcholine, and/or norepinephrine (Schultz, 2015; Holly & Miczek, 2016; Durschmid, Zaehle, Hinrichs, Heinze, Voges, Garrido, et al., 2016; Takahashi, Langdon, Niv, & Schoenbaum, 2016; Bunzeck, Guitart-Masip, Dolan, & Duzel, 2014; Koster, Seow, Dolan, & Duzel, 2016; Ranganath & Rainer, 2003).

Because a rewarding event is typically accompanied by an increase in dopamine in the nucleus accumbens, neuroscientists had assumed that this site mediated the "pleasure" accompanying a reward. The more likely explanation is that the rewarding event was unexpected, and this feature led to the surge of dopamine. People planning a holiday prefer to visit places they have never seen. Children who spent their first two years in an institutional setting that offered few unexpected experiences are usually retarded in select cognitive abilities (Nelson, Fox, & Zeanah, 2014). It is possible that the primate brain requires a minimal level of unpredictability early in life in order to establish the connections necessary for normal development.

Chimpanzees who find a dead member of their group in the forest behave as if they are surprised rather than sad (van Leeuwen, Mulenga, Bodamer, & Cronin, 2016). A border collie had been trained over many years to associate each of 200 spoken words with 200 different objects. On hearing an unfamiliar word, which was unexpected, the animal retrieved the only unfamiliar object in a room containing seven familiar objects

(Kaminski, Call, & Fischer, 2004). Even the tiny brain of the locust responds to an unexpected change in the path of a moving stimulus (Bockhorst & Himberg, 2015).

One-year-old infants who expect a woman in a video clip to move her hand in a particular way and to follow a particular path show distinctive reactions when the woman's identity, the form of her movement, or the path is altered (Song, Pruden, Golinkoff, & Hirsh-Pasek, 2016). Sleeping newborns respond to the less frequent sound in an oddball paradigm, defined by many presentations of one stimulus and a small proportion of another (for example, a ratio of 80 to 20) (Haden, Nemeth, Torok, Dravucz, & Winkler, 2013). Some four-month-old infants staring at a schematic face covering a speaker baffle will cry when they hear a human voice coming from the speaker because this event violates their expectation of seeing a person nearby (Kagan & Snidman, 2004). The emergence of crying in response to a stranger as well as to the mother's departure in an unfamiliar place, two phenomena that emerge between 7 and 12 months, are due to the infant's inability to assimilate these unexpected events. Adults from one of six cultures describing the events that are the usual origins of each of seven emotions agreed that an unexpected experience was the most common incentive for fear (Scherer, 1997). These events are also the bases for the most vivid childhood memories (Rubin & Kozin, 1984).

Although the hippocampus typically reacts to unexpected events, the class of event has implications for the brain profile. For example, among adults reading nouns that belong to a particular semantic category, an unexpected change in the font of the letters activated the fusiform region. A change in the semantic category was accompanied by activation of the inferior prefrontal cortex. A change in the valence of the word from pleasant to aversive led to increased blood flow to the amygdala (Strange & Dolan, 2001).

The relation between the magnitude of deviation from the expected and the magnitude of the behavioral response often assumes an inverted U-shaped function. I noted earlier that infants devote their longest bouts of attention to events that share some, but not all, of the features of a familiar, expected stimulus (Godard, Baudouin, Schaal, & Durand, 2016; Kagan, 1970, 1994). Selective attention to stories in newspapers follows a similar function (Teigen, 1985). An unexpected event has to engage some representation in order to provoke increased attention (Kumaran & Maguire, 2007).

More than 70 years ago Hebb (1946) noted that captive chimpanzees were most likely to show behavioral signs of fear to objects that shared some features with their knowledge (a human head, skull, and monkey). The animals displayed minimal fear to objects that shared few or no features with their acquired representations (a wooden bug, mechanical grasshopper, and small grub). (See Forss, Schuppli, Haiden, Zweifel, & van Schaik, 2015 for a similar result.) Eight-year-old children honor this principle. They display larger P3b waveforms to the spoken name of a friend or their own name than to the names of strangers because the former, although unexpected, engaged their knowledge (Key, Jones, & Peters, 2016).

Many patients with obsessive-compulsive disorder experience an uncomfortable tension when they detect a slight deviation from their understanding of how an object or scene should appear or how an action should feel. One woman reported this feeling when her memory of the way she placed a letter in a mail box moments earlier did not match her expectation of how she expected to feel (Coles & Ravid, 2016)

Volunteers for a psychological study who are not told what they will see do not expect the examiner to show them pictures of violence, sex, blood, or diseased bodies. As a result these scenes activate the amygdala because one of its primary functions is to respond to an unexpected event, whether desirable or threatening (Comte, Schon, Coull, Reynaud, Khalfa, Belzeaux, et al., 2016; Balderston, Schultz, Hopkins, & Helmstetter, 2015; Ferretti, Caulo, Del Gratta, Di Matteo, Merla, Montorsi, et al., 2005; Koh, Wilkins, & Bernstein, 2003; Davis & Whalen, 2001; Jaaskelainen, Pajula, Tohka, Lee, Kuo, & Lin, 2016; Sarinopoulos, Grupe, Mackiewicz, Herrington, Lor, Steege, & Nitschke, 2010). The amygdala's response to pictures of snakes with open jaws or revolvers reflects surprise rather than fear or anxiety when these sights are unexpected (Davis, Neta, Kim, Moran, & Whalen, 2016; Amado, Hermann, Kovacs, Grotheer, Vidnyanszky, & Kovacs, 2016; Jocham, Brodersen, Constantinescu, Kahn, Ianni, Walton, et al., 2016; Pape, 2005). The brain and behavioral response to an unexpected event is muted when the animal or person can anticipate its occurrence (Rekkas & Constable, 2006). Adults listening to sequences in which the fifth sound was always different from the prior four did not display the usual MMN waveform because they could anticipate the less frequent event (Sussman, Chen, Sussman-Fort, & Dinces, 2014). The screams of bonobo chimpanzees who are victims of an unexpected attack differ from the screams that accompany an expected attack (Clay, Ravaux, de Waal, & Zuberbuhler, 2016).

The evidence is overwhelmingly persuasive of the conclusion that unexpected events, whether neutral, desired, or aversive, activate the amygdala of animals and humans (McHugh, Barkus, Huber, Capitao, Lima, Lowry, & Bannerman, 2014; Williams,

Oler, Fox, McFarlin, Rogers, Jesson, et al., 2015; Vrticka, Lordier, Bediou, & Sander, 2014; Balderston, Schultz, & Helmstetter, 2011; Belova, Paton, Morrison, & Salzman, 2007; Nishijo, Ono, & Nishino, 1988; Amaral & Adolphs, 2016). Despite these facts, some investigators continue to insist that an increase in amygdala activity to unexpected pictures or words classified, a priori, as threats reflects fear or anxiety rather than surprise (Shackman & Fox, 2016). If the published studies of the brain profiles recorded to such threats were repeated with subjects who knew what they would experience, I suspect the results would be seriously different.

I make this suggestion because a meta-analysis of the BOLD signals to the conditioned stimuli (CS+) used in Pavlovian fear conditioning with humans revealed increases in blood flow to the anterior insula, ventral striatum, somatosensory region, prefrontal cortex, and cerebellum, but not to the amygdala because the CS+ ceased to be a surprise after the initial trials (Fullana, Harrison, Soriano-Mas, Vervliet, Cardoner, Avila-Parcet, & Radua, 2016; Wendt, Schmidt, Lotze, & Hamm, 2012; Holland & Schiffino, 2016).

The social behaviors of pairs of macaque monkeys, familiar with each other and interacting in a familiar place, are also inconsistent with the hypothesis that activation of the basolateral and central nuclei of the amygdala reflects a fear state. Temporary chemical activation of either site did not generate actions signifying fear. Rather, activation of the basolateral area led to a small decrease in requests for grooming from the other member of the dyad, and social behaviors were unchanged when the central nucleus was activated (Wellman, Forcelli, Aguilar, & Malkova, 2016). These results are consistent with the absence of fearlessness in adult monkeys whose amygdalae had been lesioned at birth (Moado, Bliss-Moreau, & Amaral, 2015). It is worth noting that the basolateral region is proportionately larger in humans than in apes, but humans are less fearful to strangers and unfamiliar settings than apes (Barger, Stefanacci, & Semendeferi, 2007). This fact implies that this site is biologically prepared to respond to any unexpected experience.

Kinds of Uncertainty

The brain and psychological states generated by an unexpected event depend on its desirability and familiarity. An unexpected gift from a friend could be familiar (a scarf) or unfamiliar (a container for coins made of tree bark). An unexpected but unwanted event could be familiar (a cold after a year free of any illness) or unfamiliar (a package containing a small skull). Although investigators often use the term *uncertainty* as if it described a single state, there are at least four kinds of uncertainty (Kagan, 2009).

An unexpected event creates stimulus uncertainty, which is often accompanied by increased gamma band activity in the frontal lobe, and activation of the amygdala and frontal cortex (Durschmid, Edwards, Reichert, Dewar, Hinrichs, Heinze, et al., 2016; Wetzel, Buttelmann, Schnieler, & Widmann, 2016).

The state created by an inability to predict what might occur in the next moment, hour, or day is a second type of uncertainty. This state has no consensual name in English, but the thoughts and feelings implied by the German word *angst* come close to capturing this subjective state (Wierzbicka, 1999).

Events or settings that activate more than one possible response, as well as those for which the agent has no response, create a state called response uncertainty (Catena, Perales,

Megias, Candido, Jara, & Maldonado, 2012). A driver in an unfamiliar region who confronts a choice of three roads with no sign is in this state. The ventral striatum is activated when an animal or person is unsure of the most appropriate response in an ambiguous situation (Haber, 2016). The central gray is activated when individuals are unsure of how to respond to an imminent pain of unknown intensity (Yoshida, Seymour, Koltzenburg, & Dolan, 2013).

Conceptual uncertainty, probably restricted to humans, emerges when a person cannot resolve an inconsistency between or among their semantic networks. American women conversing with Asians speaking with a Southern accent showed an increase in heart rate because of the inconsistency between their categories for ethnicity and accent (Mendes, Blascovich, Hunter, Lickel, & Jost, 2007). Adults reading semantically incongruent noun-adjective pairs, such as "yellow zebra" and "wrinkled lamp," displayed large BOLD signals that were absent when they read congruent pairs like "yellow banana" and "shiny lamp" (Reggev, Bein, & Maril, 2016).

Words can evoke associations that render a sentence incongruent. Although sentences ending with an incongruent word are usually accompanied by an N400 waveform because they are unexpected, the magnitude of the waveform is smaller if the incongruent word has an association with another word in the sentence. The expected word *guitar* in the sentences, "The counselor strummed as we sang by the campfire. Everyone loved the sound of his guitar" did not produce an N400. Although replacing *guitar* with the words *clarinet* or *sparks* rendered the second sentence equally incongruent, these terms evoked a smaller N400 than the word *book* because the former are associates of words in one of the sentences. *Clarinet* is an associate of *sound* and *sparks* an associate of *campfire* (Amsel, DeLong, & Kutas, 2015; Metusalem, Kutas, Urbach, & Elman, 2016).

A small proportion of adults automatically see a color when they hear or read a word, a phenomenon called synesthesia. Among some adults in this group, certain phonemes evoke a color. One such adult saw brown when she heard words beginning with *d* because the sound triggered an association to dogs and subsequently the color brown. Another saw green to the word Saturday because it began with the letter *s*, which is a salient phoneme in the word grass (Miozzo & Laeng, 2016).

Many significant scientific discoveries began with an unexpected observation that evoked conceptual uncertainty. Francois Jacob was surprised by the delay in the growth of a colony of bacteria when he added a second sugar to the food source. Ernest Rutherford did not expect to observe particles aimed at a gold sheet to be deflected. Charles Darwin was puzzled by the variation in the carapaces of the tortoises on different islands in the Galapagos chain. It takes a prepared mind to recognize the significance of an unexpected observation. The hired assistants who gather the primary data in large laboratories are unlikely to apprehend the significance of an observation that violates consensual theory.

Children as young as age four experience conceptual uncertainty when their belief in a proportional relation between events is violated. Children recognize that the magnitude of most outcomes is proportional to the force applied, whether the distance a ball moves when thrown, the pain felt when struck with a large versus a small object, or the sound made by a large versus a small object when it falls on a hard surface. These experiences, and others, lead them to expect a proportional relation between the severity of a punishment and the seriousness of the transgression and between the amount of reward a child should receive for participation in a task and the effort or talent applied to the endeavor.

Contemporary Americans are not angered by all instances of income inequality. They are especially peeved by inequalities that fail to honor proportionality. They do not object to the high incomes of talented athletes, singers, surgeons, inventors, or film stars because these adults worked hard to exploit a special talent. Many do resent the extraordinary incomes of those who work in the financial industry because they believe these men and women did not possess a special talent and took advantage of contacts that a majority could not access. Hence, their wealth was gained unfairly.

Adults who are betrayed by a friend, lover, or spouse are liable to become intensely angry. Those who were betrayed by a member of the clergy are vulnerable to a blend of anger, guilt, and anxiety (Flynn, 2008). Anger is also common among those who believe that their current life circumstances are unfair. A much smaller group is susceptible to guilt, rather than anger, if they believe that they are partially responsible for a traumatic experience, such as being a victim of rape, war, or a robbery (Stotz, Elbert, Muller, & Schauer, 2015; Nishith, Nixon, & Resick, 2005).

Many biblical scholars believe that the emphasis in the Old Testament on guilt and gaining the knowledge needed to be obedient to God represents the wish by the authors to remind the Hebrews, who had returned to Palestine by 520 BCE to form a coherent society, that the sins of their ancestors, not lack of bravery or a weak military, were the reason why the Babylonians had destroyed the Temple in Jerusalem in 586 BCE. The exile of Adam and Eve and the destructive flood that saved only Noah and his passengers were intended as warnings to the new generations of Hebrews to follow the Laws in order to avoid future catastrophes.

A small proportion of survivors of concentration camps, massacres, or natural catastrophes are susceptible to guilt if they believe they did not deserve to escape harm. If their private answer to the query, "Why me?" is that their personal traits, accomplishments, or morality were no different from those who perished, their privileged state seems unfair and a violation of the principle of proportionality (Weisz, 2015; Trappler, Cohen, & Tulloo, 2007; Trinh, Nadler, Shie, Fregni, Gilman, Ryan, & Schneider, 2014; Zhang, Duan, Xu, Jia, Bai, & Liu, et al., 2015; Thoresen, Jensen, Wentzel-Larsen, & Dyb, 2016).

Muslim youth who identify with their religious group, are a distinct minority in their community, and also enjoy the material advantages of an affluent family, are susceptible to guilt over the stark contrast between their comfortable lives and the conditions of the many poor or displaced Muslims in Iraq, Afghanistan, and Syria. This combination renders them receptive to radicalization by ISIS or another Islamic group. The *New York Times* of April 10, 2016, described such a young man who was caught by the FBI as he prepared to fly to the Middle East to join ISIS.

Hope of Success

All successful therapies for a mental illness possess some unexpected features that clients associate with the therapy's effectiveness. About one-third of depressed patients given a pill they believed would mute their melancholic mood reported significant improvement, even though the pill was a placebo

(Furakawa, Cipriani, Atkinson, Leucht, Ogawa, Takeshima et al., 2016). Psychoanalysts require patients to lie on a couch and free-associate. This form of therapy was successful for about 50 years. After the rituals had lost their novelty, both clients and analysts lost some faith in the curative power of the procedure. The rituals of psychoanalytic therapy are novel to contemporary Chinese, and wealthy Chinese are seeking this form of therapy. Cognitive behavioral therapy (CBT) has been a popular treatment for depression for about the same length of time. Recent evaluations, however, reveal that it is no more or less effective than any form of dynamic psychotherapy with an experienced therapist (Gibbons, Gallop, Thompson, Luther, Crits-Christoph, Jacobs, et al., 2016).

Most individuals who believe that a novel ritual will alleviate their distress usually report a benevolent outcome. Middle-class Swedish women who worried excessively about odd bodily sensations they did not understand were treated, over a 12-week period, with either a set of pamphlets to read or on-line conversations with a therapist. Both groups showed equivalent improvement because both expected their therapy to be helpful (Hedman, Axelsson, Andersson, Lekander & Ljotsson, 2016).

Expectations of success or failure exert a significant influence on the decision to invest effort in attaining a goal, whether an exam grade, a term paper, a relationship, a therapy, or a career. The unpleasant feelings that accompany failure are usually more intrusive than the pleasure that comes with success. The anticipation of shame or guilt after a failure often dwarfs the expectation of pride that would follow a successful effort. As a result, most youth and adults need to believe that success is possible if they try to attain it. This phenomenon also honors an inverted

U-shaped function. Effort is maximal when the person is just a little unsure of victory.

Teachers who have low expectations for the progress of their black or Hispanic pupils from poor families are less likely to invest the effort needed to facilitate their progress. The children, in turn, do not develop the expectation that they will acquire the skills needed for admission to a college or pursuit of a gratifying career. Youths from families where one or both parents are professionals have an important advantage. Their identification with their family persuades them that they probably possess the talent to attain a similar goal.

The capacity to anticipate events in the distant future is the foundation of the remarkable perseverance humans display in the face of repeated frustrations. Hundreds of thousands of scientists are working 80-hour weeks in the hope of making a discovery that will last for at least their lifetimes. Their persistence, despite the low probability of success, implies that the experiences accompanying pursuit of the goal are the source of the pleasure.

Experiences that violate firmly entrenched expectations can alter—sometimes in a moment—the quality of an emotional relationship that has lasted for years. Arthur Miller captured this phenomenon in *Death of a Salesman*, in the scene where Biff discovers the father he idealized in a hotel room with a prostitute. An experience on an autumn afternoon in 1941, when I was 12 years old, altered my conception of my father, and, later, led to a questioning of all authority. The day was Yom Kippur and at breakfast my father and I declared our intention to honor the imperative to fast until sundown. Around two o'clock in the afternoon, after the morning service was over, I was walking on a street in the small town where we lived. As I looked down the street toward a bakery my father frequented, I saw the owner and my father leaving the shop eating buns. At that moment my unquestioning respect for the declarations of authority dissolved. I owe my father a debt of gratitude. The skeptical frame that emerged that afternoon has been an important ally in my research and has affected my reflective evaluations of the conclusions reached by other scientists.

4 Sources of Evidence

Bohr's insightful proposal that the validity of a statement about nature depends on its source of evidence resolved a controversy over whether light was a wave or a particle because the outcome of directing photons toward two narrow slits depended on whether scientists did or did not try to measure each photon's path. The same principle applies to conclusions about brain and behavior. The validity of a statement is distinct from its meaning. Meaning, as Wittgenstein proposed, rests with a language community's consensual understanding of a sentence. A shared understanding, however, does not guarantee that the events described have been or could ever be observed. Catholic scholars have a consensual understanding of the meaning of statements about the Resurrection; string theory physicists have a shared meaning of multiple universes. These agreements do not guarantee that the Resurrection occurred or that multiple universes exist. It is useful to distinguish among the validity of a statement about nature that is based on certain observations, the truth of a conclusion that is based on the coherence of a logical or mathematical argument, and the rightness of a moral proposition based on a feeling.

The popular way to phrase Bohr's principle is to write that scientists assign a probability to the validity of each statement in accord with the evidence cited to support it. Statements that refer to exactly the same observation can have more than one validity if they are based on different evidence. The validity of the sentence "Snow is white" spoken by a person who has seen snow differs from the validity of the same statement made by a blind adult who has neither seen snow nor read or heard of its color, but explains that she guessed its white color from its temperature.

The validity of Newton's prediction that the world would last until 2060, based on his reading of Revelation, differs from the validity of the same prediction made by contemporary physicists who rely on different evidence, even though both predictions are likely to be affirmed (Grayling, 2016). Newton was right for the wrong reasons, but the reasons award special validity to a statement.

Bohr's position differs from the view of a number of philosophers who argue that a statement is valid if it corresponds to the way things are in nature. But the way things are in nature is not obvious when the phenomena are not observable directly and have to be inferred from theoretically expected outcomes of hypothetical entities. Conclusions about brain chemistry provide an example. Some scientists infer the tonic level of dopamine in the striatum from the frequency of spontaneous eye blinks because D2 receptors in the striatum mediate this response and Parkinson's patients, who have low levels of dopamine in this site, display reduced rates of eye blinks. This rationale was called into question recently by the observation that stimulation of D2 receptors with a drug had no effect on blinking (Jongkees & Calzato, 2016).

The diverse psychological processes that define the concept called Theory of Mind must also be inferred from indirect evidence. Children's answers to the false belief test are regarded as an index of one component of a Theory of Mind. The child must infer that person A will go to the place where she had placed an object, rather than to a second location where another adult had moved it without A's knowledge after A left the room. Although two-year-olds can infer that an adult needs help or is in pain, most children do not pass the false belief test until they are four years old because a correct reply requires not only the ability to infer the thoughts of another, but also an understanding of the meaning of the question being asked, especially the term *where,* and the capacity to inhibit the urge to point to the second, displayed location when the examiner asks where A will look for the object. The latter two talents show major improvement between the third and fourth birthdays (Espy, 2016). The claim by Setoh, Scott, and Baillargeon (2016) that two-year-olds can pass the false belief test was based on a change in the evidence. Specifically, the second agent removed the object from the room, rather than place it in the second location when A was absent. Because this procedural change removed the need to inhibit the urge to point to the last location where the children saw the object, it altered the evidence used for the earlier claim that young children fail the false belief test.

Earlier research with nonhuman primates that also used a voluntary behavior revealed that apes fail the false belief test. The investigators eager to prove that apes possess an element of Theory of Mind had to use a very different kind of evidence. They measured the brief, involuntary saccades that apes made to each of the two locations (Krupenye, Kano, Hirata,Call, & Tomasello, 2016). Because there were more saccades to the location where A had hidden the object, they suggested that apes passed the false belief test.

However, this result could reflect the fact that the first event in many, non-painful sequences is often the most salient and best remembered. The first word in a list of 12 words is often the one most likely to be recalled. The events of the first day on a college campus are usually better remembered years later than the events of the last day. Although the saccade evidence is seriously different from the voluntary actions of four-year-old children, the investigators who want to believe that apes possess a Theory of Mind ignore that fact. Studies that support a popular assumption are more often published and cited than those that challenge a majority opinion (deVries, Roest, Franzen, Munafo, & Bastiaansen, 2016). The many nineteenth-century psychologists who were certain that the young infant's behavior contained elements of adult traits were receptive to the declaration that the newborn's reflex closing of the fingers on a pencil placed on the palm was an early sign of adult greed. The discussion that follows accepts Bohr's principle that the validity of every conclusion depends on the observations that a particular procedure generated. In this frame, validity is a property of statements inferred from a specific kind of evidence.

The Role of Theory

Scientists rely on agreement with consensual theory to decide on the evidence that awards a particular statement a privileged validity. This strategy is easier to apply in physics, chemistry, and biology, which have some sound theoretical principles, than in the social sciences where there is minimal consensus on theory.

Bartoshuk (2014) provides a particularly persuasive demonstration of Bohr's position and the role of theory. When adults who varied in the number of taste buds for sweetness judged a sip of soda on a scale that went from "Not sweet" to "Very sweet," those with many taste buds gave the same judgments as those with fewer receptors. This result implies the counterintuitive conclusion that the sensation of sweetness is unrelated to the number of receptors for this quality. However, when the same adults were asked to adjust a lever controlling the loudness of a sound so that the perceived intensity corresponded to the intensity of sweetness of the soda, those with more taste buds selected a loudness value resembling a train whistle; whereas those with fewer taste buds selected the sound of a dial tone. The answer to the question "Do individuals with more taste buds for sweetness experience a given food as sweeter than those with fewer taste buds?" is "It depends on the evidence." (See Forkmann, Scherer, Meessen, Michal, Schachinger, Vogele, & Schulz, 2016 for a similar result involving detecting one's heartbeats.)

One interpretation of Bartoshuk's observations is that the words describing variation in sweetness did not evoke a subtle change in feeling, but the variation in loudness did (Wang, Wang, & Spence, 2016). Very loud sounds and extremely sweet tastes generate an unpleasant feeling. Moderately sweet tastes and soft sounds evoke a pleasant feeling. Adults find it easier to match tastes to sounds than to words because both tastes and sounds evoke feelings that invite similar evaluations. Hence, theory favors the validity of the conclusion that relied on the variation in sound level. Individuals recalling a memory evoked by a cue usually selected an earlier experience when an odor, rather than a word or picture, was the evocative cue because the odor generated a feeling (Willander & Larsson, 2006; see also Koppel, & Rubin, 2016). Because feelings are often evoked by the sounds of the words that bilingual adults learned during childhood, compared with the words in their second language, swearing and decisions involving risk or the morality of an action are affected by the language in which the problem is posed (Hayakawa, Costa, Foucart, & Keyser, 2016).

The validities of the declarations about autism have changed dramatically over the past 75 years because both evidence and theory were altered. The initial claim that the cause of the disorder, whose prevalence 70 years ago was one in every 2500 American children, was an emotionally detached mother—often called a refrigerator mother—was based on the inferences of physicians interviewing and observing the personalities of parents in an office setting. The current evidence, which includes behavioral observations, analyses of brains and genomes, along with parents' descriptions, indicates that the prevalence of autism, now renamed the autistic spectrum, has increased to one in every 68 children (Vogel & La Salle, 2016). The validity of the currently high estimate is traceable to the reliance on evidence that earlier investigators never included.

Because the definition of posttraumatic stress disorder (PTSD) in the DSM-5 manual, published in 2013, modified the definition in DSM-IV, the validity of some conclusions about this illness published after 2013 have also changed (Hoge, Yehuda, Castro, McFarlane, Vermetten, Jetly, et al., 2016). Kenneth Kendler (2016) is justifiably bothered by the fact that some clinicians who use only DSM criteria when diagnosing depression ignore salient symptoms that patients report. This fact means that scientists performing meta-analyses on this illness category are analyzing heterogeneous sources of evidence and will arrive at conclusions with different validities. Clinicians would award some patients different diagnoses if they interviewed them on two separate occasions, which they rarely do, because many report different symptoms when interviewed a second time (Chmielewski, Clark, Bagby, & Watson, 2015).

Test scores, parent reports, and observations on monozygotic (MZ) and dizygotic (DZ) twin pairs furnished the values in the equations that estimated the heritability of psychological traits. These equations assumed identical levels of expression of the genes possessed by an MZ twin pair. Recent evidence revealing differences in gene expression in MZ siblings, due partly to variation in epigenetic marks, challenges the earlier theoretical premise and alters the validity of the initial estimates of heritability.

The validity of conclusions about the memory deficiencies of H.M., who had large sections of his temporal lobe removed to reduce his seizures, depended on the procedure. H.M.'s ability to remember a particular picture he had seen six months earlier was close to that of normal adults when the picture was presented along with one he had not seen. But his memory was impaired when he saw only a single picture and had to say whether he had seen it in the past (Freed & Corkin, 1988). The procedure that allowed him to compare old with new helped him retrieve his knowledge. That is why students prefer true–false questions to those asking for definitions of concepts or essays.

Although a majority of studies of infant cognition rely only on changes in total time looking at an event that violates an expectation, investigators who record the longest fixation or the number of shifts in the focus of attention often arrive at conclusions that differ from those based solely on total time looking (Courage, Reynolds, & Richards, 2006). Failure to display an increase in total looking time does not always mean that the infant did not detect a change in a stimulus (Keating & Keating, 1993).

Technology and New Evidence

The invention of an instrument that generates new observations often alters the validity of older beliefs. Galileo's telescope allowed him to see details on the moon that challenged the idea that God made the heaven's objects free of imperfections. The introduction of new machines that record the variation in temperature and the density of energy across the universe has led to a small crisis in astrophysics (Clark, 2016; Gribbin, 2016). The evidence generated by the Wilkinson Microwave Anisotropy Probe, which measures energy density, invites conclusions different from those implied by the data produced by the Planck space probe, which measures the variation in microwave radiation across the cosmos. The small temperature fluctuations in space are inconsistent with the standard model cosmologists have relied on for many years.

Peter Galison (1997) documents a major change in physics in the 1970s when many scientists replaced the evidence that came from studying observable phenomena, such as the orbit of a planet or the track of a particle in a Wilson cloud chamber, with computer programs that analyzed large numbers of values, some hypothetical, in order to arrive at conclusions about events or entities that were difficult to imagine. The Big Bang, the Higgs boson, and the temperature of the oceans or earth 200,000 years ago are examples. The development of the camera in the 1830s, which allowed investigators to photograph faces with varied expressions, altered the validity of certain statements about emotions (Pichel, 2016). Francis Galton's invention in the 1870s of a procedure that made composite photographs of the faces of many adults provoked discussion of the typical face of a murderer or rapist (Sera-Shriar, 2015). In the same century, the invention of the stereoscope and tachistoscope stimulated research on visual illusions which challenged the validity of the traditional premise that the senses registered reality accurately (Schurer, 2016).

Brain–Behavior Dissociations

The introduction of fMRI scanners, magnetoencephalography, and powerful amplifiers for neuronal signals have had profound effects on the validity of statements about psychological phenomena. The literature is replete with conclusions about a relation between brain and psychological evidence whose validity varies with the evidence (Fischer, Luaute, & Morlet, 2010; Desmurget, Reilly, Richard, Szathmari, Mottolese, & Sirigu, 2009; Rajalingham, Stacey, Tsoulfas, & Musallam, 2014).

More than 30 years ago a team of investigators argued that brain activity preceded a person's conscious intention to act. This conclusion was based on a change in the electroencephalogram, called the readiness potential, which occurs about 350 msec before subjects report an intention to act (Libet, Gleason, Wright, & Pearl, 1983). These scientists assumed that an intention to act was a discrete point in time, rather than a process, and that the verbal report of intention corresponded to the time when the intention occurred. Investigators relying on different evidence for intention concluded that the readiness potential did not occur earlier than the intention to act (Matsuhashi & Hallett, 2008; Verbaarschot, Haselager, & Farquhar, 2016).

Psychological observations of a woman who was unresponsive for five months following an accident revealed no evidence of consciousness. However, brain measures invited a different conclusion, for the woman displayed an increase in blood flow to the supplementary motor cortex when an examiner asked her to imagine playing tennis (Owen, Coleman, Boly, Davis, Laureys, & Pickard, 2006). Women suffering from excessive constriction of the muscles of the pelvic floor find sexual intercourse painful. Although some of these women said they regarded the sexual act as disgusting, they did not show distinctive BOLD signals to scenes illustrating explicit sexual activity (Borg, Georgiadis, Renken, Spoelstra, Weijmar-Schultz, & de Jong, 2014).

Scientists who had observed a few individuals born without a corpus callosum wrote that anyone lacking this structure would show impaired motor behavior and speech. But recent work has revealed that some children born with complete agenesis of the corpus callosum fail to show any obvious delay in motor function or speech (Al-Hashim, Blaser, Raybaud, & MacGregor, 2016).

The magnitude of the negative waveform in the EEG between 250 and 300 msec following brief exposures to snakes, spiders, beetles, and worms were larger in response to snakes than to spiders, implying a stronger emotional response to snakes. But most of the participants displaying these large waveforms rated the spiders as more frightening than the snakes (Van Strien, Christiaans, Franken, & Huijding, 2016).

Investigations of humans using the technologies of fMRI and magnetoencephalography (MEG) occasionally arrive at slightly different conclusions (Garces, Pereda, Hernandez-Tamames, Del-Pozo, Maestu, & Angel Pineda-Pardo, 2016; Winterer, Carver, Musso, Mattay, Weinberger, & Coppola, 2007). This is not surprising because the two procedures reflect different processes quantified with distinctive metrics.

The BOLD signals that emerge from changes in oxygenated blood to varied sites reflect the proportional decrease in deoxygenated hemoglobin in the veins proximal to the sites of neuronal activity and are a more accurate index of the neuronal activity created by synaptic inputs to a cell, measured as local field potentials, than neuronal spiking rates (Kim & Ress, 2016; Driver, Andoh, Blockley, Franklin, Gowland, & Paus, 2015; Denfield, Fahey, Reimer, & Tolias, 2016).

The BOLD signal in a 1.5 Tesla scanner has relatively good spatial resolution, between 1 and 3 mm^3, but poor temporal resolution, about 3 sec at best (Buxton, 2013). However, the spatial resolution is not good enough to capture variation in activity in the grid cells of the entorhinal cortex when adults are imagining moving in space to a location (Horner, Bisby, Zotow, Bush, & Burgess, 2016). Nor are these signals able to detect differential activity in the core and shell of the nucleus accumbens, in each of the three regions of the medial orbitofrontal cortex (Dreyer, Vander Weele, Lovic, & Arogona, 2016; Henssen, Zilles, Polonero-Gallagher, Schleicher, Mohlberg, Gerboga, et al., 2016), or the different areas of the intraparietal sulcus (Zlatkina & Petrides, 2014).

It is also relevant that the magnitude of change in the BOLD signal is affected by small movements, eye blinks, muscle tension, respiration, diameter of the veins, and cardiovascular events that have a minimal effect on most behaviors (Reuter, Tisdall, Qureshi, Buckner, van der Kouwe, & Fischi, 2015; Nakano, Kato, Morito, Itoi, & Kitazawa, 2013; Driver, Andoh, Blockley, Francis, Gowland, & Paus, 2015; Potts & Mitchell, 1998; Macefield & Henderson, 2016).

In addition, a half-second after each systole, neural activity in the form of an event-related potential, called the heartbeat evoked potential (HEP), is recorded in several brain sites (Taggart, Sutton, Groves, Holdright, Bradbury, Brill, & Critchley, 2007). The variation in the magnitude of the HEP is likely to be accompanied by different BOLD signals and, in some cases, by a subtle change in the quality of consciousness (Park, Bernasconi, Bello-Ruiz, Pfeiffer, Salomon, & Blanke, 2016). Subjects with a high heart rate should display a different pattern of BOLD signals than those with a low heart rate, even though their cognitive functions may be equivalent (Salomon, Ronchi, Donz, Bello-Ruiz, Herbelin, Martet, et al., 2016). Inferences from BOLD data are also influenced by whether the analysis is performed on single voxels or patterns of voxels, called MVPA. Although the latter have become popular, conclusions can depend on whether the investigator does or does not ignore the direction of change in the BOLD signals (Gilron, Rosenblatt, Poldrack, & Mukamel, 2016).

Magnetoencephalography (MEG), on the other hand, measures the magnetic field generated by current flow in the dendrites of a large number of neurons (at least 50,000) located in sulci that are tangential to the scalp. MEG data have better temporal resolution, but poorer spatial resolution, than blood flow. The MEG signal is larger when a regular pattern of tones becomes random; whereas the BOLD signal is greater when a random pattern of tones becomes regular (Barascud, Pearce, Griffiths, Friston, & Chait, 2016). Many adults display slightly different MEG and BOLD patterns to pictures of objects, actions, and gratings (Swettenham, Muthukumaraswamy, & Singh, 2013).

The validities of conclusions based on relations between the magnitudes of the BOLD signals to the amygdala, especially the lateral nucleus, and a subsequent psychological state vary because the distinctive projections from the lateral amygdala generate different evidence. The ventral amygdalofugal pathway projects to sites in the striatum that are responsible for motor responses, such as flight. The bed nucleus of the stria terminalis, on the other hand, projects to sites in the hypothalamus that activate the HPA axis and sympathetic targets to produce different measurements (Kamali, Sair, Blitz, Riascos, Mirbagheri, Keser, & Hasan, 2016; Oler, Tromp, Fox, Kovner, Davidson, Alexander, et al., 2016). When an animal must make an active avoidant response in order to avoid electric shock, for example move to a different location or strike a lever, the central nucleus is inhibited so that freezing will not occur, while the projections from the basal nucleus to the nucleus accumbens are enhanced so that the active avoidance response is possible (LeDoux, Moscarello, Sears, & Campese, 2016).

The dissociations between the inferences drawn from brain or psychological data are occasionally due to the fact that sites which make no important contribution to the psychological outcome show increased activity (Mur, Ruff, Bodurka, Bandettini, & Kriegeskorte, 2010). Subjects who are anxious in the scanner are apt to activate sympathetic targets, which lead to activation of the insular cortex. It would be an error to conclude that the insula made an essential contribution to the perception of motion in subjects who felt unsure of their ability to deal with the task.

The BOLD signals in occipital, parietal, and temporal cortex in adults reading a prose passage one word at a time overlapped substantially with the patterns recorded to a wedge moving across the visual field, meaningless vocal sounds, and movements of different parts of the body (for example, wrinkling the eyebrows, touching a thumb, or moving a toe) (Sood & Sereno, 2016). This fact implies that some of the activated sites were not essential contributors to the process being studied. Buxton (2013) has suggested that arterial spin labeling (ASL) should be added to the BOLD signal in order to arrive at more valid conclusions. Although ASL provides a more accurate index of the perfusion of a site, it has a poor signal to noise ratio and its use constrains the number of images that can be taken in a short interval.

The practice of basing inferences on the difference between the pattern of blood flow to an event of interest and the pattern to a baseline event poses a serious problem because the choice of baseline event is critical to the conclusion (Buxton, 2013). Subjects with unusually low baseline BOLD signals are likely to show larger increases to an incentive than those with high baselines (He, 2013). This phenomenon, called the Law of Initial Values, applies to many variables, including ERP waveforms (Bradford, Kaye, & Curtin, 2014; Meyer, Lerner, De Los Reyes, Laird, & Hajcak, 2017). If I compare the weight of 10 oranges using 10 lemons as the baseline, I will conclude that oranges are heavier. But if I compare the weight of 10 oranges with 10 watermelons I will conclude that oranges are lighter.

Many psychologists believe that a potentiated eyeblink reflex to a brief burst of loud sound while individuals are exposed to an unpleasant event is a valid measure of fear or anxiety because most adults display a larger startle to the loud sound when they are looking at unpleasant, compared with pleasant or neutral, scenes. But the latter two kinds of scenes are inappropriate baseline events because most subjects do not expect to see pictures of bloodied bodies, angry faces, or rotted food but are more prepared to see the familiar scenes of an infant, an apple, or a chair.

Hence, the unpleasant pictures recruit more focused attention, which, in turn, enhances the magnitude of the eye blink startle (Bradley, Lang, & Cuthbert, 1993). College students solving anagram problems or suddenly plunged into darkness show potentiated startles, but do not report feeling anxious while solving the problems or sitting in the dark (Sorenson, McManis, & Kagan, 2002; Grillon, Merikangas, Dierker, Snidman, Arriaga, Kagan, et al., 1999).

Adults in a virtual reality setting who had earlier been familiarized with the distinctive features of two rooms received unpleasant air puffs to the toe or finger in only one of the rooms. In a subsequent phase they were exposed to a third room which contained a few features that were present in each of the two earlier rooms. Although the subjects rated their level of anxiety higher in this third room than in the safe location where they were not shocked, the magnitude of potentiated startle was similar to the level recorded in the safe room (Andreatta, Leombruni, Glotzbach-Schoon, Pauli, & Muhlberger, 2015). Because there is no consensus on the meaning of an enhanced startle, it is difficult to determine anxiety level from startle evidence.

The blending of the brain's responses to the phases of a cascade that ends with a perception, thought, feeling, or action poses a frustration to investigators deciding on the conclusion to infer from brain data (Morris, Bremmer, & Krekelberg, 2016). Neuronal profiles in occipital regions V1, V2, and V3, which are responsive to the directions and locations of contours in the visual field, blend with later activity in the lateral occipital cortex, which is tuned to specific features of an object (Vernon, Gouws, Lawrence, Wade, & Morland, 2016).

Cascades involving thalamic nuclei are especially important because of reciprocal connections between these nuclei and varied cortical sites. The occurrence of a saccade is preceded by a cascade involving at least six brain sites (Hallock, Wang, Griffin, 2016; Vertes, Linley, & Hoover, 2015; John, Zikopoulos, Bullock, & Barbas, 2016). The response of lateral geniculate neurons to the enhanced contour contrast in the enlarged eyes of a fearful facial expression is a major determinant of the activation of the amygdala and visual cortex. The peak BOLD signals to a site, recorded several seconds after an incentive appeared, is a blend of a cascade of events that began during the initial 100 msec (Mc Garry & Carter, 2016; Freiwald, Duchaine, & Yovel, 2016; Jones, Fontanini, Sadacca, Miller, & Katz, 2007).

Brain Measures of Concepts

A number of scientists believe it is possible to localize a semantic concept in a particular site or circuit. This hope deserves some scrutiny because the structures of concepts change with time and experience. Semantic concepts are usually defined as networks of connected hubs containing schemata and semantic representations that share one or more features. The hubs activated in a person hearing, reading, or thinking about a particular exemplar of a concept depend on the setting. Hammers and wine openers are both exemplars of the semantic concept *tools*. But the names of these objects are members of other conceptual networks. Hammers are members of the network for carpenters and wine openers belong to the network for dinner parties. This claim implies that most semantic concepts are not localized in a single site or circuit. Rather, the neuronal ensemble activated by a term depends on the hubs that were primed by the thoughts that the local circumstances evoked.

It appears that the validity of statements describing the properties of a concept depends on whether brain or psychological evidence is cited. A multidimensional scaling of the features that adults assigned to exemplars of the concepts fruits, vegetables, vehicles, tools, mammals, birds, natural scenes, and artificial places revealed two dimensions. One reflected the symbolic contrast between animate and inanimate objects; the other contrasted foods with locations. However, a multidimensional scaling of the voxels that generated the largest BOLD signals revealed a different pair of dimensions. The first contrasted animals, which have curved contours, with places, which have more linear contours. The second dimension contrasted small with large objects as they appeared in the world. More relevant is the observation that the voxels that best differentiated among the eight concepts were located in the parietal and occipital lobes, which respond to an object's physical features and locations, rather than sites in the anterior temporal lobe, which react to semantic meanings (Handjaras, Ricciardi, Leo, Lenci, Cechetti, Cosottini, Marotta, & Pietrina, 2016). The brain and psychological evidence invite different inferences about the primary features of these concepts.

Current brain measures fail to reveal a number of abstract concepts that every person possesses. This statement applies especially to the concepts *good* and *bad*. Adult judgments of the good examples of a semantic category, compared with the bad ones, did not correspond to any profile of BOLD signals because the latter were unduly influenced by the physical features in the scenes, rather than the goodness of the example (Torralbo, Walther, Chai, Caddigan, Fei-Fei, & Beck, 2013).

More than 50 years ago Osgood, Suci, and Tannenbaum (1957) asked adults from a large number of cultures speaking different languages to rate words referring to categories of people, animals, or objects on ordinal scales marked at each end by a member of an antonym pair (for example, active–passive, slow–fast, big–small, good–bad, sweet–sour, high–low, light–dark). A factor analysis of the ratings revealed that most subjects, across the cultures, relied implicitly on the contrast between the semantic concepts good and bad as the primary determinant of their judgments. This dimension, which psychologists call valence, contrasts pleasant with unpleasant feelings and moral with immoral actions and people.

Had investigators measured the brains of these adults as they rated the words it is unlikely that the resulting patterns would have revealed the implicit reliance on the concepts good and bad because of the heterogeneity in the physical features of the exemplars of the concepts. Although the concepts of good and bad represent a primary hub in human semantic networks, they do not appear to be a primary basis for brain profiles recorded up to now. That is why there are no distinctive BOLD signals to paintings judged as ugly (Kawabata & Zeki, 2004).

Potency, a second dimension that emerged from the adult ratings, would also be hidden in brain evidence. Size, strength, force, speed, status, resistance to alteration, and a capacity to alter conditions are primary properties of potent objects, people, animals, or events (Kagan, Hosken, & Watson, 1961). The Chinese scholar Lao Tzu, in the fifth century BC, wrote, "Sweetest of all things is this: the power each day to seize what one most wants."

Children, as well as adults, relied on a potency dimension when they selected the most appropriate sentence, from pairs of sentences with the same literal meaning. In the following examples a majority selected the sentence in which the less potent object was mentioned first as the more appropriate. "The fire hydrant is close to the building" was favored over "The building is close to the fire hydrant." "South Korea is like China" was chosen over "China is like South Korea," and "My sister met Barack Obama" was selected over "Barack Obama met my sister" (Chestnut & Markman, 2016).

One reason why brain measures would have failed to reveal the potency dimension is that the more potent alternative is always relative to the comparison being made. Adults who regard a building as more potent than a fire hydrant would judge the building as less potent if it were next to an airport, and regard the airport as less potent if it were next to a large body of water. Evaluations of valence are less susceptible to the specific comparison being made. A sweet taste, a caress, an act of kindness, and a correct answer to a problem are classified as good across diverse comparisons. Visiting a friend who is ill does not lose its status as a good act because donating an organ to save the friend's life is an even kinder act.

Physical Features of Events

Although valence and potency are primary features of psychological networks, the brain is sensitive to the physical features of events. This fact helps to explain the differential validities of statements about mental processes based on brain compared with psychological evidence, especially conclusions about the structures of concepts. Although scientists would like to believe that the brain profile evoked by a meaningful picture or word reflects mainly the processing of its acquired meaning, the physical features of the stimulus generate an initial wave of activity in many sites that is independent of the event's meaning

(Izquierdo, Furini, & Myskiw, 2016; El-Shamayleh & Pasupathy, 2016). The features in visual events, which are studied more often than other modalities, include the linearity, curvature, orientation, and symmetry of contours, luminance contrasts, spatial and radial frequency, wavelength, motion, and location in the visual field. Neurons in the parahippocampal place area are tuned to respond to linear contours that form right angles (Nasr, Echavarria, & Tootell, 2014). The lateral occipital cortex is more responsive to convex than to concave contours (Haushofer, Baker, Livingstone, & Kanwisher, 2008). My brain responds to a single white spot moving slowly on a blue-green surface at least a fifth of a second before I recognize a sailboat on a smooth sea. Neurons in the superior colliculus respond faster to stimuli in the upper half, compared with the lower half, of the visual field (Hafed & Chen, 2016). The features that define long, coiled objects, characteristic of hoses, balls of string, cables, and snakes, activate the superior colliculus, pulvinar, and amygdala when they fall on the fovea (Almeida, Soares, & Castelo-Branco, 2015). Neurons in the cat's primary visual cortex respond more to a moving dark bar on a light background than to a light bar on a dark background (Kremkow, Jin, Wang, & Alonso, 2016).

Because the brain can respond to the separate features of an object, it is not always possible to predict the neural response to the whole pattern from the response to its elements. For example, there is maximal neuronal activity in posterior cortex to a square containing a vertical line inside and a vertical line below. But there is no activity to the same square containing the line below, but missing the inside line (Gilbert, 2012). Adults have no trouble recognizing a face in a drawing in which two wine-glasses replace the eyes. Although. a normal face evokes an N170 waveform in the EEG, this slightly altered face does not (Bentin, Golland, Flevaris, Robertson, & Moscovitch, 2006).

The pattern of spatial frequencies in the stimulus is always important. Some adults experience a mildly aversive feeling to events that combine high-contour contrast with mid-range spatial frequencies. A dark hole on a sunny day and honeycombs are two examples (Cole & Wilkins, 2013). The right hemisphere is receptive to lower spatial frequencies and the left is preferentially responsive to higher spatial frequencies (Rajimehr, Devaney, Bilenko, Young, & Tootell, 2011). Experienced radiologists rely on the higher spatial frequencies in breast X-rays to detect cancerous tissue, which they can do in less than a half-second (Evans, Haygood, Cooper, Culpan, & Wolfe, 2016).

Neurons in the dorsal stream are preferentially tuned to lower spatial frequencies but higher temporal frequencies. Neurons in the ventral stream are tuned to both high and low spatial frequencies, but smaller temporal frequencies (Canario, Jorge, Silva, Soares, & Castelo-Branco, 2016; Kristensen, Garcea, Mahon, & Almeida, 2016).

Because the right hemisphere is especially receptive to lower spatial frequencies, neurons in the monkey's right amygdala are activated by the eyes in faces with fearful expressions (Montes-Lourido, Bermudez, Romero, & Vicente, 2016; Hedger, Adams, and Garner, 2015; Caldera, Seghier, Rossion, Lazeyras, Michel, & Hauert, 2006). The variation in the spatial frequencies of more than a thousand pictures of humans, animals, natural objects, or artifacts explained more of the variation in the BOLD signals to the parahippocampal place area, retrosplenial complex, and occipital place area than the object's semantic category (Lescroart, Stansbury, & Gallant, 2015). This observation is consistent with the fact that the patterns of BOLD signals in the ventral stream to pictures of intact bottles, chairs, faces, houses, and shoes resembled the patterns recorded to scrambled versions of the same pictures whose semantic category was unrecognized. This evidence implies that the physical features of the objects had a greater influence on the brain profile than their semantic category (Cogan, Liu, Baker, & Andrews, 2016). (See Bracci & de Beeck, 2016 and Haxby, Connolly, & Guntopalli, 2014 for similar results.) In light of the evidence, it is not surprising that a computer analysis of the contour junctions, angles, orientations, and curvature of line drawings made from color photographs of beaches, forests, mountains, city streets, highways, and offices was as accurate as human judgments in assigning each photo to its proper semantic category (Walther & Shen, 2014). The brain's reactions to the physical features in a scene contribute to the remarkable accuracy of four-year-olds in detecting whether one object is inside, on top of, under, or in front of another (Farran & Atkinson, 2016).

The BOLD signal to the intraparietal sulcus when subjects are exposed to different numbers of black dots has been interpreted as reflecting the processing of the number of dots. However, the number of dots is correlated with the circumference of the array and/or the size or density of the dots and, therefore, the dominant spatial frequency of the array (Dakin, Tibber, Greenwood, Kingdom, & Morgan, 2011).

The BOLD signals to the posterior superior temporal sulcus of adults looking at more than a thousand faces displaying one of seven emotions were best interpreted as responses to the physical features in the faces (for example, large eyes, open mouth, wrinkled forehead, or a raised upper lip) rather than to the emotion represented (Srinivasan, Golomb, & Martinez, 2016). Adults detect facial expressions of happiness at very low levels of emotional intensity because these faces combine the presence of teeth without closed eyes. This is not true of anger, sadness, fear, disgust, or surprise (Calvo, Avero, Fernandez-Martin, & Recio, 2016). Investigators who claim that each basic emotion is instantiated in a specific blood flow profile are ignoring the influence of the physical features of the faces symbolic of fear, anger, joy, sadness, surprise, or disgust (Saarimaki, Gotsopoulos, Jaaskelainen, Lampinen, Vuilleumier, Hari, et al., 2016; Srihasam, Vincent, & Livingstone, 2014; Van Renswoude, Johnson, Raijmakers, & Visser, 2016).

One pair of psychologists argued that seven-month-old infants could detect trustworthiness in faces because they looked longer at male faces adults had judged as trustworthy compared with untrustworthy (Jessen & Grossmann, 2016). However, the mouth area in the untrustworthy faces was turned down, as in a frown. The trustworthy faces did not contain this feature. It is likely that the infants' looking behavior was guided by this variation in physical features rather than by a judgment of trustworthiness.

The pictures classified as unpleasant, pleasant, or neutral in many studies of the brain's response to emotional incentives are not perfectly matched for physical features. Revolvers, teeth, spiders, broken objects, a truck in a ditch, and a tank with an artillery gun are likely to have one or more angular contours. Pleasant pictures, such as smiling infants, ice cream, and sex scenes, are more likely to have curved contours and fewer angles. The amygdala is more responsive to events containing angular, rather than curved, versions of the same neutral objects (Bar & Neta, 2007).

Eyes regularly activate a number of brain sites, including the amygdala, especially when they fall on the fovea (Mosher, Zimmerman, & Gothard, 2014). The wide eyes in fearful facial expressions activate the amygdala 70 msec before neurons in the prefrontal cortex respond (Luo, Holroyd, Jones, Hendler, & Blair, 2007). A pair of wide eyes characteristic of a fear face without any other facial features, activates the right amygdala when presented for only 17 msec and followed by a neutral face as masking stimulus (Whalen, Kagan, Cook, Davis, Kim, Polis, et al., 2004; Kim, Solomon, Neta, Davis, Oler, Mazzulla, & Whalen, 2016). A cortically blind adult with bilateral destruction of the primary visual cortex showed amygdalar activity to a face with a direct gaze (Burra, Hervais-Adelman, Kerzel, Tamietto, de Gelder, & Pegna, 2013). Monkeys whose amygdalae had been lesioned soon after birth showed more prolonged freezing to a human intruder looking at them directly than when the adult looked away (Bachevalier, Sanchez, Raper, Stephens, & Wallen, 2016).

Epileptic patients with electrodes implanted in the amygdala saw a face with a neutral expression morph over a half-second into a happy or a fearful face that was either staring at them or looking away. The faces that stared at the viewers, happy as well as fearful, evoked the largest ERP waveforms, despite the fact that they represented different emotions, because of the presence of the eyes in the direct gaze (Huijgen, Dinkelacker, Lachat, Yahia-Cherif, El Karoui, Lemarechal, et al., 2015). Infants look a little longer at a monkey's face containing human eyes rather than the animal's eyes because of their larger sclera and greater contour contrast (Dupierrix, de Boisferon, Meary, Lee, Quinn, Di Giorgio, et al., 2014).

Punctate versus Gradual Events

The brain is sensitive to the duration of a stimulus and the time it takes to reach peak intensity, called rise time. Punctate events have shorter durations and more rapid rise times. Gradual events have the opposite set of features. A punctate or gradual stimulus in one sensory modality is likely to be associated with the same property in another modality. A light that attains high intensity quickly is treated as similar to the sound of a fire alarm.

A picket fence, the smell of sulfur, the taste of mint, the voiceless consonants *k*, *p*, and *t*, the vowels *e* and *i*, and the nonsense words *queek*, *takete*, and *kiki* are more punctate than a ball, the smell of a rose, the taste of a banana, the consonants *b*, *m*, *n*, the vowels *o*, *a*, *u*, and the nonsense words *bouba*, *maluma*, and *toota* (Koppensteiner, Stephan, & Jaschke, 2016; Sidhu & Pexman, 2015). American children as young as age three associate the vowels *a*, *o*, and *u* with round shapes and the vowels *e* and *i* with angles (Maurer, Pathman, & Mondloch, 2006).

Punctate sounds are more likely to have a higher pitch than gradual ones, and higher-pitch sounds are associated with thinness, speed, a lighter weight, brightness, and unpleasant events (Walker, 2016). Laughter is one exception to the last claim. Spontaneous, involuntary laughs have a higher pitch, but a longer duration, than faked laughs. People use this blend to detect the difference between the two kinds of laughs (Lavan, Scott, & McGettigan, 2016).

American and British parents are biased to choose a name with punctate features for their sons and a name with gradual properties for their daughters. The five most popular names for girls in 2015 end in a gradual vowel: Sophia, Emma, Olivia, Ava, and Mia. The popular names for boys—Jack, Jacob, Thomas, George, and William—end in a punctate consonant (Pitcher, Mesoudi, & McElligott, 2013; Wright, 2006).

The Effect of Effort

Scientists who study relations between the brain and a psychological outcome often ignore the influence of the mental effort participants invest in meeting an examiner's request. The requirement to perform a task necessarily affects the pattern of blood flow and the more difficult the task, the greater the effect on BOLD signals (Egidi & Caramazza, 2016). Adults had to pick the one word from a trio that was most closely related to a probe word. The trio always contained one word that belonged to the same conceptual category as the probe and one word that had a relational link to the probe. If the probe was *dog* the conceptual match might be *cat* and the relational word *bone*. Although linguists regard this distinction as important, and children shift from relational associations (*dog–bone* or *dog–bark*) to conceptual associations (*dog–cat* or *dog–horse*) by age seven, the magnitude of the BOLD signals was determined mainly by the difficulty of the particular trio of words, rather than by this linguistic distinction (Jackson, Hoffman, Pobric, & Lambon-Ralph, 2015).

The effort needed to assimilate a sentence or the final word of a sentence can influence activity in select temporal lobe neurons that is independent of the activity that reflects the processing of meaning (Fedorenko, Scott, Brunner, Coon, Pritchett, Schalk, & Kanwisher, 2016). The effect of effort is seen in a study in which adults silently read sentences that varied in the frequency, length, and predictability of the words. The magnitude of the BOLD signal to temporal and frontal sites was smaller to sentences containing more frequent, predictable words because these sentences were easier to comprehend (Schuster, Hawelka, Hutzler, Kronbichler, & Richlan, 2016; see Parkes, Perry, & Goodin, 2016 for another example). One reason why symmetrical arrays of elements are more pleasing, and generate brain responses different from asymmetrical ones, is that the former require less effort to process.

Music students singing consonant and dissonant intervals displayed greater activation in many sites to the latter intervals because they are more difficult to sing (Gonzalez-Garcia, Gonzalez, & Rendon, 2016). Activity in the dorsolateral striatum of rats trained to make the correct turn in a T-maze to receive a reward declined as the correct response became automatic in over-trained animals (Smith & Graybiel, 2016; see Huddleston & DeYoe, 2008, and Fischer, Mikhael, & Kanwisher, 2016 for other examples of the relation between effort and brain response). The evidence implies that the neural activity accompanying the investment of effort is blended with the activity reflecting the processing of the psychological meanings of the incentive or the implementation of a response (Salamone, Correa, Farrar, & Mingote, 2007).

The Influence of Associations

The BOLD signal is also affected by the subject's associations, sometimes idiosyncratic, to the event (Kleint, Wittchen, & Lueken, 2015). Dutch adults selecting the two words from a triad of semantically unrelated terms that were most closely related relied primarily on a shared location or function, taxonomic category, or part of a whole and secondarily on valence or a lexical feature as the bases for their choices (De Deyne, Navarro, Perfors, & Storms, 2016). Given the triad car, carnation, and rat one could rely on the function of motion and pick words one and three, rely on the category natural object and select the second and third terms, or select the first two words because they begin with the same letter. The important point is that the adults found it easy to detect a property shared by a pair of unrelated words, although they did not always agree on the shared property for a particular triad.

Investigators who record the BOLD signal to the angular gyrus in adults looking at the face of a famous actress cannot be sure whether this site is responding to the shape of her face, her name, the title of one of her films, or scenes from the films in which she played a leading role (Bar, Aminoff, & Ishai, 2008). Italians, and perhaps others as well, acquire associations between the color yellow and triangles and between red and circles (Albertazzi, Da Pos, Canal, Micciolo, Malfatti, & Vescovi, 2013). Italian students possess associations between the concept of sacredness and shapes that have either vertical or curved contours (Costa & Bonetti, 2016).

Nouns associated with actions, such as *hand, foot,* or *tongue,* excite sites in motor cortex that in some instances make no contribution to the comprehension of the word's meaning (Bonner, Peelle, Cook, & Grossman, 2013). The patterns of activity in the occipitotemporal cortex of adults looking at parts of the human body implied the evocation of associations representing the function of that part (Bracci, Caramazza, & Peelen, 2015). Adults looking at pictures they had seen during the prior three weeks displayed BOLD signals to so many brain sites it was impossible to know which activations represented the schema or semantic label for the scene and which were elicited by associations (Rissman, Chow, Reggente, & Wagner, 2016; see Morel, Beaucousin, Perrin, & George, 2012; Heisz & Shedden, 2009; Gobbin & Haxby, 2006, for additional examples of the influence of associations on brain profiles). The main point is that investigators are vulnerable to misinterpreting the meaning of an activated site in a subject who had idiosyncratic associations to an incentive.

A review of 57 studies of multivoxel pattern analysis (MVPA) invited two major conclusions. First, frontal, temporal, and parietal sites were activated by such a variety of incentives and tasks it was difficult if not impossible to be certain of the appropriate inference to be drawn. Second, although activations of motor, visual, or auditory cortex usually corresponded to the incentive, there were instances when a profile of activation did not match the input (Woolgar, Jackson, & Duncan, 2016).

The complete corpus of evidence has prompted some neuroscientists to question the practice of treating brain measures as sensitive proxies for psychological processes, especially thoughts, emotions, and beliefs (Poldrack & Yarkoni, 2016; Weinberger and Radulescu, 2016; Eysel, 2003). Their skeptical evaluation is reasonable, given the fact that the brain's reaction to an incentive is influenced by the context, the collection of events, the subject's expectations, effort, associations, and the specific measure of brain activity. It is unlikely that the brain state that accompanies seeing a picture of a snake on a screen while lying in a scanner would resemble the pattern actualized when the same person, hiking in a fall forest, sees a similar looking snake while hearing the sounds of birds, looking at colorful leaves, and coordinating limb movements on a deeply rutted trail.

The Denial of Mental States

Most neuroscientists are suspicious of conclusions that award a causal power to mental events that transcends the material processes from which they emerged. This conviction was held by nineteenth-century investigators hoping to establish a materialistic account of behaviors based on learned associations. The Russian physiologist I.M. Sechenov claimed that a thought was the final phase of an inhibited reflex (Smith, 1992). Freud borrowed this premise when he posited the concept of sublimation.

The rejection of any view of mind that retained the tiniest trace of dualism is one reason why Tolman's research in the 1930s was not awarded the significance it deserved (Tolman, 1932, 1938). Scientists studying psychiatric disorders are fond of the phrase, "Mental illnesses are diseases of the brain." This assumption ignores the contribution of thoughts and emotions to every mental illness. The authors of an otherwise insightful essay on the need to replace current psychiatric categories with symptoms emphasized only the biological contributions and omitted references to the beliefs that childhood histories created (Gillan & Daw, 2016). Experts studying obesity do not declare that excess weight is a disease of the fat cells because they recognize the contributions of improper eating habits.

The popularity of the idea that mirror neurons are the foundation of understanding, despite evidence inconsistent with this claim, is due in no small measure to the desire to retain a materialistic basis for thought (Rizzolatti & Craighero, 2004). This hypothesis assumed an earlier form in the writings of Silvan Tomkins (1962, 1963) who suggested that the neural signals from facial muscles to brain were the origin of an emotional experience.

However, it is the person's interpretation of the feelings that arise from bodily activity that determine the emotional state and any actions that follow. A child's interpretation of the feelings generated by a parent's abuse, or an adult's reinterpretation of an earlier abuse, is a more critical determinant of the probability of developing pathology than the objective fact of having been abused (Luke & Banerjee, 2013). The importance of interpretations explains why religious Israelis from settlements near the Gaza Strip subject to terrorist attacks reported fewer symptoms than secular Jews residing in the same dangerous settlements (Kaplan, Matar, Kamin, Sadan, & Cohen, 2005).

The failure of BOLD signals to anterior cortical sites to differentiate between the psychological state of an operatic star listening to recordings of her voice compared with recordings of another woman singing similar songs, even though the woman must have had self-referential thoughts while hearing herself sing, points to the special properties of thought (Zaytseva, Gutyrchik, Bao, Poppel, Han, Northoff, et al., 2014).

Beliefs

Beliefs are an important set of mental events that have causal power. Among the many beliefs that children and adults establish, one kind has distinctive properties. This class of beliefs links membership in a family, class, community, ethnic, religious, or national category with the potential for an emotional experience. These beliefs, called identifications, combine representations of the distinctive features shared by both the person and another with the experience of vicarious emotions appropriate to the other that influence the judgment of self's valence and potency. The vicarious emotion that is an essential element in an identification has to be distinguished from an empathic feeling or thought. Most individuals who feel empathy for a dog in pain or Syrian refugees do not believe that they share distinctive properties with these victims. Therefore, their empathy does not have a powerful influence on the private evaluation of their personhood.

The establishment of an identification requires a number of inferences. Young children automatically treat different objects that have the same name as members of a common category (Waxman & Braun, 2005; Ferry, Hespos, & Waxman, 2010). When children learn that they share the same surname with one or both parents and any siblings they infer that they and the other members of their family belong to a common category.

By the fifth or sixth birthday children assume that objects belonging to the same category share properties that they have not observed (Carey, 2009). If they learn that all living things called animals feel pain and sleep, it is reasonable to assume that an unfamiliar form, say an octopus, that is labeled an animal must also feel pain and sleep. This reasoning implies that children who know that they and one or both parents possess the same surname, skin color, and the material substances transmitted to them at conception and during gestation, will infer that they probably share other qualities they have not observed. A seven-year-old daughter of a mother who is a well-known writer may assume that she possesses the potential to be as talented as her parent.

The phenomenon of vicarious affect rests on a pair of different mechanisms. Children older than five or six can imagine how others, friends as well as strangers, might evaluate a member of their family who had done something that ought to be praised or condemned. This ability is a component of the stage of concrete operations (Piaget, 1950). Children now assume that others are likely to evaluate them with the same judgment they impose on the parent. This thought is usually accompanied by either vicarious pride or shame.

The second mechanism is revealed in research demonstrating that the brain sites activated when a monkey executes a motor action are activated when the animal sees another monkey perform the same response. This phenomenon, also observed in humans, was initially attributed to neurons in an area of the frontal lobe called mirror neurons (Rizzolatti & Craighero. 2004). Although later research has questioned the validity of the earlier claim that these mirror neurons were needed to understand the action, this phenomenon has relevance for vicarious emotion (Hickok, 2014; Rizzolatti & Sinigaglia, 2016).

The mirror neuron evidence implies the ease with which any member of an acquired association can activate the other. Listening to the heart beats of another person activates the same sites in insular cortex as hearing one's own heart beats (Kleint, Wittchen, & Luecken, 2015). Watching another receive a tactile stimulus activates sites in the sensorimotor cortex of the observer (Lankinen, Smeds, Tikka, Pihko, Hari, & Koskinen, 2016). These facts imply that a boy who learns that his father is depressed because he lost his job is apt to activate the brain sites that were aroused on the past occasions when he felt sad. As a result, the son, too, will experience a vicarious sadness.

Vicarious pride is also common. Amos Oz, a celebrated Israeli author, remembered the emotion he felt the day his father, also a respected writer, told his six-year-old son he could place his childhood books on the same shelf that held the father's volumes. Michael MacDonald, born to a poor Irish family in South Boston, recalled the vicarious pride in his national-ethnic group when the residents of his Irish neighborhood resisted a judge's decision to bus Irish children to schools in distant neighborhoods in the service of desegregating the city's public schools (MacDonald, 1999).

Youth are most likely to acquire identifications with their ethnic, religious, social class, or national group when the group possesses distinctive features in the society. This process can be observed in a laboratory. Five-year-olds assigned to one of two arbitrary groups showed facial and postural signs of guilt when a member of their group committed a transgression (Over, Vaish, & Tomasello, 2016).

An identification with one's family pedigree is, for most youth and adults, the strongest. Patrick Modiano, the 2014 Nobel Laureate in Literature, titled his 2015 memoir *Pedigree* because he wanted his readers to know the vicarious shame he felt as the son of two marginalized, irresponsible adults in post-war France. Modiano wrote, "That's the soil—or the dung—from which I emerged."

Vicarious guilt can be intense when a family member violates a significant moral imperative. Rainer Hoess was a happy, confident, twelve-year-old who was unaware that his deceased grandfather, whom he never knew, had been a Commandant at Auschwitz. Soon after he learned this disturbing fact, Rainer sank into a serious depression because this knowledge implied that he, too, might have some of the properties of a cruel killer.

Each person continually surveys their networks in search of inconsistencies in the valence or potency of the exemplars. An adolescent who learns that her mother is a drug addict confronts an inconsistency in her network for the parent that she attempts to repair by altering the nodes responsible for the inconsistency. Success is not guaranteed if the valence of a node resists alteration (Cao & Banaji, 2016). Rainer Hoess's depression illustrates this resistance.

Although a few studies find reasonable changes in brain patterns when a person experiences a vicarious emotion, more data are needed (Mobbs, Yu, Meyer, Passamonti, Seymour, Calder, et al., 2009; Vachon-Presseau, Roy, Martel, Albouy, Chen, Budell, et al., 2012; Singer, Seymour, O'Doherty, Kaube, Dolan, & Frith, 2004).

Most investigators ignore the causal power of mental events, including the consequences of identifications, for at least four reasons. First, thoughts and feelings are difficult to measure, can last for a brief interval, and cannot be easily parsed into separate elements. Thoughts and feelings vary in valence, referents, duration, and intrusiveness, which subjects can rate reliably. However, feelings also vary in qualities that are much harder to quantify because of the absence of words to describe them. The available candidates are fuzzy terms such as vital, aroused, vigilant, relaxed, irritable, and serene. One reason for the sparse vocabulary is that the bodily sites that give rise to feelings do not possess as rich a set of receptors as vision, hearing, smell, taste, and touch. Children and adults with a more active viscera are susceptible to the intrusiveness of feelings they often interpret as worry, tension, or uncertainty. Those with a hypoactive viscera are vulnerable to a feeling tone they interpret as apathy (Owens, Low, Iodice, Critchley, & Mathias, 2016).

Individuals use the thoughts evoked by a setting to decide on the emotional term that is the best interpretation of the intrusiveness and quality of their feeling (Fox & Beevers, 2016). Consider a woman who experiences a sharp rise in arousal when she cannot open the door of her bedroom in order to leave the room. Initially, she selects surprise as the term to describe her state, but quickly shifts to fear when the door does not yield to her continued action and she cannot explain why. Seconds later the woman decides she is angry when she hears her son's movements in the hall and suspects he locked her in the room. The woman's brain state at this moment is a blend of the profiles of neuronal activity that were the foundations of the changes in her feelings and interpretations.

The resistance to acknowledging that a mental event that emerged from one brain state can influence subsequent brain profiles, bodily events, and psychological processes is inconsistent with evidence. Adults with a cast covering their forearm and hand for a month were able to retard the loss of muscle strength by imagining they were flexing these muscles (Clark, Mahato, Nakazawa, Law, & Thomas, 2014). The establishment of a memory for a movement is facilitated when the agent plans the movement ahead of time (Sheehan & Franklin, 2016).

A parent who made sense of the death of a child was less likely to develop a serious depression than one who could not create an explanation that removed all personal responsibility for the tragic event (Keesee, Currier, & Neimeyer, 2008). The interpretation that Chinese adolescents imposed on the feelings evoked by exposure to the severe earthquake of May 12, 2008, affected the probability of developing the symptoms of posttraumatic stress disorder (Wang, Long, Li, & Armour, 2011). The level of activity in the insular cortex to pictures of dirty toilets and corpses was reduced in women who believed that the pill they had ingested would decrease feelings of disgust (Schienle, Ubels, Schongasner, Ille, & Scharmuller, 2013). The fact that the brains of men and women react differently to the intranasal administration of oxytocin or vasopressin attests to the power of thought, because men and women interpret the feelings these molecules create in different ways. The BOLD pattern recorded in women imagining a dildo stimulating their genitals was absent when they imagined a physician's speculum touching the same tissues (Rilling, Demarco, Hackett, Chen, Gautam, Stair, et al., 2014; Scheele,

Striepens, Kendrick, Schwering, Noelle, Wille, et al., 2014; Chen, Hackett, DeMarco, Feng, Stair, Haroon, et al., 2015; Wise, Frangos, & Komisaruk, 2016).

A person's conscious intentions or future plans affect their brain profiles (Einhauser, Rutishauser, & Koch, 2008; Quellet, Santiago, Funes, & Lupianez, 2010). Individuals preparing for sleep try to decrease their level of arousal. Those preparing for an examination seek to maximize their alertness. A combination of 38 biological measures gathered on more than a thousand adults who slept in their own bed was a poor predictor of each person's subjective judgment in the morning of how well they had slept (Kaplan, Hirshman, Hernandez, Stefanicki, Hoffman, Redline, et al., 2016). Although almost everyone wants others in their community to judge them favorably, no scientist has found a brain profile that represents that wish or generated it with optogenetic methods.

Why the Resistance?

The reluctance to acknowledge that a thought originating in one brain profile could generate a new brain state is sustained, in part, by the absence of consensual metrics for mental events. The neuroscientists' metrics of spiking rates, coherence of frequency bands, ion channels, and local field potentials are inappropriate for mental phenomena. A train of thought usually activates temporal sites that process semantic forms, parietal sites representing schemata, and frontal sites that contribute to the semantic coherence of a sequence of thoughts or sentences.

Investigators trying to discover the origin of a thought in brain activity must measure patterns of activation that involve most of the cortex. Moreover, they have to explain how continually changing brain states can be the foundation of a persistent perception or idea. This task is so daunting that many neuroscientists avoid it by not awarding mental events an autonomous causality, instead insisting they are epiphenomena. Physicists are not bothered by the fact that one class of atom can be transformed into a different atom with distinct properties, for example uranium to barium, through bombardment of the first material with neutrons. They do not regard the transformed atoms as epiphenomena.

An example of the resistance to the power of thought is seen in the papers on the origin of human morality arguing that cooperative behavior among early humans, which is observable, was a necessary predecessor to the emergence of a sense of justice and empathy (Tomasello, 2016). It is difficult to understand, however, how early humans could cooperate in hunting for large game, building a home, or caring for infants if they were unable to infer the skill, loyalty, honesty, and feelings of others.

It seems more reasonable to assume that the ability to infer another's psychological states and latent talents must have evolved before cooperation. Alfred Wallace had a similar intuition in 1864 when he wrote that unique cognitive skills were the important consequences of the evolution of the hominid brain (Eiseley, 1958). Wallace's claim is supported by the fact that apes are unable to infer the meaning of a variety of actions by members of their own species or by humans, but do display cooperative behavior (Aldridge, 2011; Tomasello, Call, & Gluckman, 1997; Volter, Sentis, & Call, 2016; Suchak, Eppley, Campbell, Feldman, Quarles, & de Waal, 2016). By contrast, eighteen-month-old children infer a variety of mental states in others before they are mature enough to cooperate with a peer in building a tower (Kagan & Herschkowitz, 2005). The ability to infer a broad range of feelings and thoughts in friends and strangers across varied settings is a uniquely human talent made possible by genes that have unique patterns of expression in the human brain (Bakken, Miller, Ding, Sunkin, Smith, Ng, et al., 2016).

The reluctance to acknowledge the emergence of novel thoughts is reminiscent of the premise held by many eighteenth century, European scholars that all knowledge must have an origin in sensory experience. The fact that a two-year-old who has never looked for a place to put the several objects he is holding will, nonetheless, open a closet door when he sees his mother approaching the door with her hands full of packages requires accepting inference as a robust phenomenon. Eighteen-month-olds will even help an adult stranger they cannot see if they infer that the adult is in need (Hepach, Haberl, Lambert, & Tomasello, 2017).

It strains credibility, at least at present, to argue that any combination of brain measures could predict the content of a novel thought that emerged without a relevant incentive in a person sitting quietly in a dimly lit room. A five-year-old being put to bed surprised his mother by asking, "How long does it take after you die before you become an angel?" It is not even possible to use a brain measure to detect when a person is lying (Meijer, Verschuere, Gamer, Merckelbach, & Ben-Shakhar, 2016). Daniel Pollen (2011), who devoted his career to research on visual perception, acknowledged how difficult it is to explain how activity in the visual cortex mediates the perception of motion, a border, or a hand.

When a brain pattern accompanies a reported or inferred thought it is not always obvious whether the thought preceded the brain profile or the brain profile preceded the thought, although neuroscientists prefer the latter causal sequence. Patients with atopic dermatitis who believed that an inert liquid applied to their forearm was an allergen reported a feeling of itching, as well as blood flow profiles that resembled the pattern recorded when a legitimate allergen was applied to the skin (Napadow, Li, Loggia, Kim, Mawla, Desbordes, et al., 2015). The three sites with the largest BOLD signals were the dorsolateral prefrontal cortex, caudate, and intraparietal cortex.

On the one hand, activity in these sites could have given rise to the report of increased itching. On the other, it is equally reasonable to argue that the person anticipated a sensation of itching (therefore activation of the dorsolateral prefrontal cortex), prepared to implement the motor acts involved in scratching the site (activation of the caudate), and imagined the location of the itching (activation of the intraparietal sulcus). The fact that neither somatosensory nor insular cortex showed large increases in the BOLD signal favors the latter explanation (See Hein, Morishima, Leiberg, Sul, & Fehr, 2016, for another example). The evidence invites acceptance of the causal role of thought in producing brain profiles that lead to psychological outcomes. It is impossible to explain why millions of men and women rise between five and six o'clock in the morning, five days a week, commute in heavy traffic more than 25 miles to a job they do not enjoy, and return at night tired and irritable without acknowledging the power of thought on human behavior. The brain states of these commuters did not force them to engage in these aversive acts. It is odd that at the same time contemporary physicists speculate about universes they cannot observe and molecular biologists write about the possible effects of pollution on epigenetic changes in the genome that they have not measured, scientists studying brain–mind relations remain loyal to Ernst Mach's principle requiring a rejection of the validity of any statement that refers to phenomena that cannot be observed directly.

Verbal Reports

Conclusions about psychological states or past experiences based only on a person's verbal descriptions possess a special validity because of their inconsistent or, in some cases, poor correspondence with behavioral or biological data. Scientists place their trust in different sources of evidence. Physicists trust mathematical arguments that explain a large corpus of data. Biologists reserve their trust for replicable observations. Many social scientists who study human traits trust the accuracy of what people say in an interview or on a questionnaire. They assume that the descriptions of habits, symptoms, moral values, emotions, or past experiences correspond closely to the evidence that would have been provided had the respondents been observed in natural settings (Clark, Listro, Lo, Durbin, Donnellan, & Neppl, 2016; Lavigne, Gouze, Hopkins, & Bryant, 2016).

Unfortunately, this optimistic premise is seriously flawed. Descriptions of psychological states, traits, beliefs, or behaviors, recent or past, do not consistently match behavioral observations, or biological measures, whether the phenomenon is how well one slept (Landry, Best, & Liu-Ambrose, 2015), executive processes (Buchanan, 2016), well-being (Wojcik, Hovasapian, Graham, Motyl, & Ditto, 2015), impulsivity (Holmes, Hollinshead, Roffman, Smoller, & Buckner, 2016), penis length (Veale, Eshkevari, Read, Miles, Troglia, Phillips, et al., 2014), abuse of cocaine (Tourangeau, 2007), maltreatment during childhood

(Scott, Smith, & Ellis, 2012), anxiety over speaking in public (Schwerdtfeger, 2004), worry about an imminent shock (Torrents-Rodas, Fullana, Bunillo, Caseras, Andian, & Torruba, 2013), self-confidence (Kimble & Seidel, 1991), symptoms of an illness (Kwan, Wojcik, Miron-Shatz, Votruba, & Olivola, 2012; or bodily sensations (Edelman & Baker, 2002). There are some exceptions. The reports of Danish adults estimating the time they were exposed to the sun during a week in the summer did correspond to the values recorded by an electronic UV-dosimeter (Koster, Sondergaard, Nielsen, Allen, Olsen, & Bentzen, 2016).

A rating of the presence or intensity of a psychological state or trait reflects the person's idiosyncratic balance among three considerations: How do I feel? How should I feel? What should I reveal to a person I do not know? The validity of statements claiming that extraversion, conscientiousness, neuroticism, openness to new ideas, and agreeableness—the so-called Big Five—are the basic human personality dimensions rests solely on replies to a questionnaire whose items originated in the English adjectives people use most often to describe others. These terms, now and in the past, refer to the traits that a person would want to know about if they anticipated interacting with a stranger. Is she sociable or restrained, hard-working or lazy, anxious or relaxed, receptive to new ideas or rigid, and easy or difficult to deal with in a time of crisis? There is no reason to assume that these traits, each with varied origins, have strong foundations in particular genes, brain states, or experiences.

The social scientists who construct items for a personality questionnaire usually rely on their intuition when deciding on the meaning that the typical respondent will infer from the question. Such intuitions are not always correct. Many years ago one of my students asked mothers who had described their three-year-old as sensitive to report their definition of this term. Some mothers said that it meant empathic; others thought it meant easily hurt; some believed it meant the potential for creativity.

The bias among many respondents to describe self or others as possessing traits that are normative and desirable in their community poses another problem (Wood & Furr, 2016). British adults with an advanced degree are most likely to live in a large metropolitan area where extraversion is valued but neuroticism is not. Thus, it is not surprising that these adults report higher levels of extraversion and less neuroticism than British adults with less education who live in smaller cities in Scotland, Wales, or the Midlands (Rentfrow, Jakela, & Lamb, 2015).

More important, different traits would emerge from a factor analysis of the behaviors of a random sample of adults observed in varied settings. Some likely dimensions are amount of physical activity outside of the workplace, talkativeness with strangers, frequency of affectionate gestures, sexual activity, smiling, frowns, conformity to authority, behavior with those of a higher status, unsolicited acts of kindness, anger outbursts, acts of physical aggression, and attempts to dominate others. It is not obvious that these 12 dimensions are less basic than the Big Five. Had Japanese psychologists invented the first personality questionnaire they would have invented items that referred to variation in the dependent relationship between individuals (student and professor or wife and husband), conformity to others, and absence of aggression in situations that invite such a response (Wierzbicka,1991).

One pair of psychologists composed a 10-item questionnaire designed to reveal variation in the preference for reappraisal, compared with suppression, of an emotion (Gross & John,

2003). The replies suggested that Caucasian women relied on reappraisal, but men preferred suppression (Spaapen, Waters, Brummer, Stopa, & Bucks, 2014). However, a person who stops to reappraise a feeling by thinking of something else (this is an item in the questionnaire) is, of course, simultaneously suppressing the feeling. The sex difference in the choice of one of these strategies may reflect a differential preference for the meaning of the words "reappraise" or "suppress." Reappraisal implies use of the mind. Suppression, on the other hand, implies action. Thoughts are reappraised but behaviors are suppressed.

Because most adults are unlikely to practice either strategy when they are happy, and would find it difficult to adopt either strategy when intensely angry, sad, guilty, or anxious, the answers to the questionnaire are likely to reflect what people think they do when they are mildly sad, angry, anxious, ashamed, or guilty. But there is no guarantee that what individuals say corresponds to what they actually do when the feelings that give rise to these emotions pierce consciousness.

Investigators who trust the accuracy of a person's memories for past events are ignoring the evidence that puts a lie to that assumption. Adults who had been interviewed 30 years earlier as high school students about school, peer, and family relationships recalled the same events. Their adult answers to select questions did not match what they had said as adolescents. For example, many who insisted having pleasant relationships with their peers reported otherwise when they were high school students (Offer, Kaiz, Howard, & Bennett, 2000).

One group of subjects was prompted at unscheduled times, seven times a day for 14 days, to report the intensity of their happiness, fear, sadness, or anger at that moment and to recall the intensity of those states at the end of each day. The correlation between the intensity of the instantaneous emotion and its intensity as reported at the end of the day averaged only 0.3 (Mik, Realo, & Allik, 2015). If the average person does not have an accurate memory of the intensity of their sadness or fear a few hours earlier, reports of the intensity of emotions experienced years earlier are likely to be seriously distorted (Kaplan, Levine, Lench, & Safer, 2016).

Close to two-thirds of New Zealand mothers whose four-year-old child had stayed in a hospital at least one night did not remember that fact when interviewed only one or two years after the hospitalization (Burakevych, McKinlay, Alsweiler, Harding, & CHYLD Study Team, 2015). If a parent cannot recall an event as emotionally salient as a hospital admission for her child, it is reasonable to suggest that the memories of 20-year-olds recalling less salient childhood events are of questionable accuracy. (See Miller, Newcorn, & Halperin, 2010; Heir, Piatigorsky, & Weisath, 2009; and Hirst, Phelps, Meskin, Vaidya, Johnson, Mitchell, et al., 2015, for additional examples.) Schacter (1999) would not be surprised by this evidence, for he has described seven kinds of errors that occur when individuals recall the past.

Other factors affect a person's reply to questions. Some informants minimize while others exaggerate the seriousness of an unpleasant experience that happened days or years earlier. Young women who reported a large number of nonfatal bodily symptoms (for example, tachycardia and difficulty breathing) exaggerated the intensity of the pain they had experienced two weeks earlier in a laboratory when they placed their hand in cold water or breathed CO_2-enriched air (Walentynowicz, Bogaerts, Van Diest, Raes, & Van den Bergh, 2015).

Most individuals exaggerate the difference between unpleasant emotions when they have to categorize them as either mild

or intense. They do not do so when rating the uncomfortable-
ness of an emotion on a five-point scale (Petersen, Schroijen,
Molders, Zenker, & Van den Bergh, 2014). Questions that imply
boys and girls are discrete categories invite respondents to exaggerate the psychological differences between the sexes. By contrast, the ratings of adults who do not know an infant's sex fail
to describe boys as more active than girls.

Questions containing abstract words often generate a broader
range of replies than those phrased with concrete terms. Americans estimating the amount of fruit in a bowl gave a broader
range of values when the abstract word *fruit*, rather than the
concrete term *blueberries*, was used (Kruger, Fiedler, Koch, &
Alves, 2014). The answers to the question, "All things considered, how satisfied are you with your life these days?" are the
bases of conclusions about subjective well-being across societies. Because the term "satisfied" is relatively abstract, it should
generate a broader range of answers than the query "All things
considered, how often over the past few months have you felt
happy with the way your life turned out?"

Adults who have not attended college are more likely to be
unsure of the meaning of a question containing one or more
abstract terms. Nonetheless, one team asked more than 900,000
adults from one of 48 nations to rate themselves, online, on a
five-point scale on a single item whose major term was suffi-
ciently abstract to invite different interpretations from such a
diverse sample. The item was: "I see myself as someone who
has high self-esteem" (Bleidorn, Arslan, Denisson, Rentfrow,
Gebaver, Potter, & Gosling, 2016).

Young adults from the United States, Brazil, China, Germany,
Poland, Ghana, Israel, and Singapore reported—usually online—
their values, the emotions they would like to experience, and

the emotions they have experienced. Although scholars familiar with these societies have described high levels of selfishness in most of these cultures, the respondents from all eight countries denied valuing self-interest, wanting to feel important, and experiencing feelings of superiority on many occasions. The majority gave politically correct, socially desirable answers to questions posed by strangers (Tamir, Schwartz, Cieciuch, Riedeger, Torres, Scollon, et al., 2016). This result is not surprising. Some adults lie to their therapists (Kottler, 2010).

The validity of conclusions about traits or past experience based on verbal reports is a serious issue when informants from language communities that do not speak English answer a questionnaire that has been translated from an original English version (Church, Alvarez, Mai, French, Katigbak, & Ortiz, 2011; Wang, 2004; Chen, Benet-Martinez, & Ng, 2014; Barger, Nabi, & Hong, 2010; Vaughn-Coaxum, Mair, & Weisz, 2016). The words selected as synonyms for the English terms often have a slightly different meaning in another language. For example, the word "fair," in a health questionnaire given to adolescents in 43 countries, was one of four possible replies to the question "Would you say your health is …? The selection of "fair" varied from 3 to 20 percent because this word did not have the same meaning across the communities (Schnohr, Gobina, Santos, Mazur, Alikasifuglu, Valimaa, & Torsheim, 2016). This problem is exacerbated when informants speak more than one language because the links to emotion are stronger in the first language a person acquired as a child (Jonczyk, Boutonnet, Musial, Hoemann, & Thierry, 2016).

Some social scientists remain unconcerned over the limited validity of inferences based on verbal replies. Adults from 10 different societies rated the immorality of harmful actions described in vignettes as either intentional or accidental. Members of two of the ten societies denied that a behavior that intentionally harmed another was more immoral than an accidental act. The investigators used this counter-intuitive observation to question the universality of the premise that all humans regard an agent's intention as a critical factor in judging the morality of a behavior (Barrett, Bolyanatz, Crittenden, Fessler, Fitzpatrick, Gurven, et al., 2016). They minimized the fact that the two deviant societies were smaller and more isolated than the others (one was in the Pacific and the other in southern Africa). More important, they did not consider the possibility that the adults from these two isolated societies were confused by a request to rate on a five-point scale the morality of an action committed by a fictional person described verbally rather than witnessed directly in a context. Under these conditions, their answers might not reflect their true beliefs. If the scientists had made direct observations of members of these two societies and noted the occasions when someone was harmed accidentally or intentionally, they would have discovered that they treated intentional and accidental acts in different ways and were far more punitive of the former behaviors. I offer this suggestion because the informants were asked to judge the morality of the outcome of a behavior, rather than the morality of the agent who caused the harm. Children and adults asked about the latter award a significance to the agent's intention that they ignore when asked about the moral status of the outcome of a behavior (Nobes, Panagiotaki, & Bartholomew, 2016). Everyone would agree that a dead infant is a bad event. But most adults, across cultures, would agree that a mother who intentionally killed her infant committed a more serious violation of a moral code than a parent who delivered a dead baby.

Parental descriptions of a child do not always correspond to observations because the social class and personality of the parent influence descriptions of their children. American mothers with less education are more likely to rate their infants as fussy than better educated parents, even though direct observations of the children do not affirm that fact (Goodnight, Donahue, Waldman, Van Hulle, Rathouz, Lahey, & D'Onofrio, 2016; see also Vaughn, Joffe, Bradley, Seifer, & Barglow, 1987). One group of parents reported the occurrence of fear, anger, or sadness in their eight-year-old twins, who were also observed at home responding to incentives designed to provoke these emotions. The parents' ratings implied that the monozygotic twin pairs were far more similar than the children's behaviors revealed (Clifford, Lemery-Chalfant, & Goldsmith, 2015).

The same is true for inhibitory control. Parental descriptions of the level of control displayed by each of their twins at two and three years of age revealed greater similarity, and therefore higher heritability values, as well as higher year-to-year stability, than observations of each child's behavior in a laboratory setting (Gagne & Saudino, 2016). Parents of identical twins rate them as more similar than direct observations reveal (Smith, Rhee, Corley, Friedman, Hewitt, & Robinson, 2013).

Although observations of children's behaviors typically reveal significant gender differences in frequency of fighting, vigorous activity, and attraction to dangerous situations, the maternal descriptions of children, given by women from 41 different countries (most had not attended high school and lived in less developed nations), failed to affirm these behavioral differences between boys and girls (Bornstein, Putnick, Lansford, Deater-Deckard, & Bradley, 2016).

The current reliance on verbal reports continues a practice that began in the 1930s with inventories designed to assess interests and personality. When the validity of such reports was questioned during the late 1940s, indirect methods such as the Thematic Apperception Test and Rorschach inkblots became popular, and remained so for about 25 years. These techniques relied on a person's words, but trained psychologists were supposed to interpret the meanings of the words.

The flaws in psychoanalytic theory that had been recognized by the 1960s turned many psychologists away from speculative inferences and toward an empiricism that accepted the evidence as it was recorded. The literal meanings of a person's statements were the bases for inferences, despite the fact that sentences are surface phenomena, whose meanings depend on the properties of the speaker and the setting. More than 90 percent of a group of 250 experts on emotion reported on a questionnaire that pride was not an emotion (Ekman, 2016). This verbal evidence does not mean that humans are unable to experience a feeling they call pride when they successfully complete a difficult task.

The habit of treating verbal reports as proxies for behavioral data poses a problem when experts want to find out if a therapy for a mental illness is helpful. The patient's subjective evaluation is usually the only evidence used in deciding whether the therapy was effective. Patients who have spent time, energy, and money and are reluctant to disappoint their friendly, supportive therapist are likely to say that they feel better, whether or not their symptoms are less intrusive. That is why placebos are often as effective as many therapies with those who have less severe symptoms. Evaluations of therapies for diabetes, cancer, or heart disease do not rely only on what a patient says about their state and always include an objective measure of a relevant biological system.

The facts invite the conclusion that the answers people give to questions posed by a stranger have a validity that is both limited to and different from the validity of conclusions based on direct observations of behavior or verbal reports combined with behavior and biology. Freud changed his theory of neurosis when he realized that many patient reports of being seduced by a parent as a child were fictions. The reification of the literal meaning of verbal reports, whether statements given by hired Mechanical Turk subjects who provide answers on-line while sitting in a room in Delhi or by members of a longitudinal sample, poses a serious problem in current research. Goethe was so despairing of the difficulty of using language to capture experience that he had his fictional hero Faust say, "No more in empty words I'll deal."

Everyone appreciates that the most detailed narrative of a soccer match, a sunset, or a suicide bomber at an airport is not a substitute for witnessing those events. A college student who reports on a questionnaire that he had a cruel father during his childhood years may believe he is telling the truth. But his belief does not guarantee that observations of the father with his young son ten years earlier would have corresponded to the verbal description. The validities of current explanations of the relations between childhood experiences and later traits assume that the early events actually occurred, not that someone said they occurred.

The constrained validity of conclusions based on a single source of evidence, whether behavior, brain data, or verbal report, implies that patterns of observations might provide statements that have a less constrained validity. The next chapter considers this suggestion.

5 Patterns

The most casual observer cannot avoid perceiving that objects are composed of patterns of elements and events consist of patterns of conditions. Many animals have bilateral or radial symmetry; many plants and land masses possess a fractal geometry. Because most biological and behavioral phenomena are the products of patterns of conditions, rather than single causes, investigators have to gather patterns of measures in order to differentiate among the varied sequences that can give rise to the same outcome. The conclusions that follow the adoption of this strategy are likely to have a privileged validity (Bizzi, Cheung, d'Avella, Saltiel, & Tresch, 2008; Logothetis, 2014). Examples are easy to find.

The correlation between the spiking rates of two neurons in primary visual cortex depends on a pattern that combines a particular stimulus with the level of attention it recruits (Ruff, & Cohen, 2016; Kohn, Coen-Cagli, Kanitscheider, & Pouget, 2016). Patterns of reciprocal excitation among thalamic nuclei, sensory cortex, vestibular cells, medial entorhinal cortex, dentate gyrus, and CA3 neurons in a rat traversing a path are the sources of activation of place cells in area CA1 of the hippocampus (Clark & Harvey, 2016; Brandon, Koenig, & Leutgeb, 2014).

Even the tame behavior of two related domesticated species can result from different patterns of gene expression. The pattern in European pigs, for example, differs from the pattern in Asian pigs (Francis, 2015; Frantz, Schraiber, Madsen, Megens, Bosse, Paudel, et al., 2015).

Eve Marder and her colleagues (Marder, 2015; Marder, 2016; Marder, Gutierrez, & Nusbaum, 2016; Gjorgjieva, Drion, & Marder, 2016) remind the neuroscientists inventing models for neuronal activity that a particular level of spiking activity can be the result of different patterns of inputs. A typical neuron receives about a thousand inputs from 100 to 300 other sites. This fact makes it difficult to be certain of the meaning of activity in a particular site (Fishell, 2016; Subramanian, Arun, Silburn, & Holstege, 2015; Tian, Huang, Cohen, Osakada, Kobak, Machens, et al., 2016). The input pattern to the nucleus accumbens, for example, determines which response, from a collection of possibilities, is most likely to occur (Floresco, 2015). The putamen and caudate nuclei rely more on proprioceptive than visual inputs during the extinction of a motor response (Goodman, Ressler, & Packard, 2016). Neuroscientists find it helpful to conceive of the brain as a collection of hubs receiving large numbers of inputs from many diverse sites and selecting outputs as a function of the pattern of incoming signals. Different patterns of inputs arriving at different hubs can generate similar outcomes. Spontaneous and conditioned eye blinks provide an example.

Patterns of Causes for Behavioral Outcomes

Most of the outcomes people care about—suicide, homicide, grade point average, anxiety, depression, drug abuse, or well-being—require patterns of conditions that include a person's biology, social class, family, school experiences, and always the cultural setting. No gene, prenatal event, or postnatal experience, considered alone, predicts any of these outcomes with a high level of confidence (Stein, Chen, Ursano, Cai, Gelertner, Heeringa, et al., 2016). A maternal infection at the beginning of the second trimester must be part of a larger pattern if it is to contribute to an impaired inability to shift attention in later childhood (Canetta, Bolkan, Padilla-Coreano, Song, Sahn, Harrison, et al., 2016). The death of a parent during childhood, which is experienced by about 4 percent of Americans before age 18, must be combined with other risk conditions in order to affect the probability of symptoms appearing at a later time (Luecken & Roubinow, 2012). The same conclusion applies to the consequences of income inequality (Lee, Marotta, Blay-Tofey, Wang, & de Bourmant, 2014) or membership in a less advantaged social class (Bekhuis, Boschloo, Rosmalen, de Boer, & Schoevers, 2016).

The children growing up on the Hawaiian island of Kauai who experienced several childhood stressors were protected from later pathology if they combined an easy-going temperament with being the only child of a younger mother (Werner & Smith, 1982; see also Musliner, Munk-Olsen, Laursen, Eaton, Zandi, & Mortensen. 2016). The victims of bullying usually possess one or more deviant traits that include a disadvantaged family, uncommon dialect, membership in an ethnic minority, poor academic performance, excessive timidity, aggressive behavior, or a physical impairment (Boden, van Stockum, Horwood, & Fergusson, 2016; Brendgen, Girard, Vitaro, Dionne, & Boivin, 2016).

The facial expressions that signal an emotion involve patterns of activity in the striated muscles (Ekman, 1992). No single muscle group (for example, the muscles that raise the brow or cause the jaw to drop) is associated with any particular emotion. The number of possible combinations of facial muscles is far larger than the number of distinct facial expressions because some patterns prevent the display of others. It is difficult to simultaneously smile broadly, open the eyes, furrow the brow, and wrinkle the nose.

Four common facial patterns form the foundation of the emotions that English calls fear, joy, sadness, anger, pride, shame, disgust, or surprise (Mehu & Scherer, 2015). Right hemisphere sites, which receive more inputs from heart, gut, lung, and muscles than do left hemisphere sites, exert greater control of the muscles of the eyes and forehead, which are prominent in anger, fear, and disgust. By contrast, left hemisphere sites exert a stronger influence on the mouth muscles that generate smiles, which are usually accompanied by less intense feelings (Muri, 2016). A large number of psychologists assume that the facial expression accompanying crying is an accurate sign of the emotional state of sadness, even though many adults cry after a victory or when welcoming home a son or daughter who has served in a war zone. Adolescents from one of the Trobriand islands interpreted the gasping facial expression that Americans treat as a sign of fear as a reflection of anger (Crivelli, Russell, Jarillo, & Fernandez-Dols, 2016).

Speech, too, requires patterns of activity in several sites. The central gray and nucleus ambiguus establish the states in glottis and thorax that generate sounds. Sites in motor cortex are required for the movements of mouth, lips, and tongue that are needed to articulate words (Holstege & Subramanian, 2016). The sound pattern in a word from a tonal language, which can have multiple meanings, combines fundamental frequency with temporal changes in frequency and loudness. The pattern in the Mandarin word *ma* determines whether the speaker intended to say mother, hemp, horse, or scold (Singh & Fu, 2016).

Patterns of Biological Measures

The experiences classified as stressors are accompanied by different patterns of physiological activity. Most events that provoke a rise in cortisol reduce the secretion of inflammatory cytokines, and vice versa (Campo, Light, O'Connor, Nakamura, Lipschitz, La Stayo, et al., 2015; Miller, Murphy, Cashman, Ma, Ma, &Cole, 2014; Shelton, Shminkey, & Groer, 2015). Because some events can be accompanied by increases in both molecules, it is useful to examine the pattern of secretions provoked by varied threats.

The balance between excitatory glutamatergic projections and inhibitory GABAergic projections creates patterns of brain activity that are correlated with different psychological outcomes (Bravo-Rivera, Diehl, Roman-Ortiz, Rodriguez-Romaguera, Rosas-Vidal, Bravo-Rivera, et al., 2015). The freezing response many animals display to a threat provides an example. In most contexts, GABAergic neurons in the ventrolateral periaqueductal gray (vlPAG) inhibit the nearby glutamatergic cells that mediate freezing. Under certain threat conditions the central nucleus of the amygdala sends GABAergic projections to the vlPAG, which suppress the GABAergic cells that had been inhibiting the glutamatergic neurons. Once released from their inhibited state, these neurons send impulses to the medulla, which in turn lead to the freezing response (Tovote, Esposito, Botta, Chaudun, Fadok, Markovic, et al., 2016). When the animal has an opportunity to learn a behavior that will prevent experiencing the aversive event, the central nucleus is suppressed, preventing freezing, and a circuit from the basal amygdala activates the nucleus accumbens (Le Doux, Moscarello, Sears, & Campese, 2016). A cascade originating in GABAergic projections from the lateral hypothalamus to the ventral tegmental area, which disinhibits the latter, is followed by increased secretion of dopamine (Nieh, Vander Wheele, Matthews, Presbrey, Wichman, Leppla, et al., 2016; Greenhouse, Noah, Maddok, & Ivry, 2016).

The levels of mRNA that transcribe the genes whose products affect GABAergic activity were measured in the right superior frontal sulcus of the postmortem brains of healthy adults as well as patients who had been diagnosed with schizophrenia, schizoaffective disorder or bipolar disorder. About one-half of the schizophrenics and schizoaffective patients, one-third of those with bipolar disorder, but only 5 percent of the controls displayed lower levels of GABAergic activity. This result points to the advantages of measuring GABAergic activity as part of a pattern of evidence when diagnosing patients who might have one of these illnesses (Volk, Sampson, Zhang, Edelson, & Lewis, 2016).

Select neurons in the cat visual cortex detect an object's direction of movement because of intra-cortical inhibition of the neurons tuned to movements in other directions (Kim & Freeman, 2016). A woman who is certain that the rose she is looking at is pink does not know that neurons in her visual cortex are suppressing the cells that generate the perception of a yellowish-red rose, while potentiating the activity of cells that lead to the perception of pink. Similarly, when the direction of movement of two moving sinusoidal gratings differs from the movement of the entire pattern (this kind of array is called a plaid), neurons in area MT inhibit the former to allow perception of the direction of movement of the whole pattern (Wang & Movshon, 2016). Before I enter my study I am equally capable of walking, running, grabbing an object, talking, singing, or sitting down and typing. Once I sit down in front of my laptop the first five responses are inhibited so that that last pair can be expressed. Current explanations of brain–behavior relations emphasize the excitatory components at the expense of the collection of inhibitory processes. Contexts select certain actions by suppressing the alternatives. The ancient Chinese scholars who believed that all phenomena were the result of a balance between the forces of yang and yin are entitled to a smile.

The slope of habituation of the brain response to an event provides information that should be combined with the mean level of activation. Adolescents who had been high-reactive infants and fearful toddlers displayed a pattern of shallower habituation and larger mean amplitude of the N400 waveform to several series of unfamiliar, but non-threatening, pictures (Kagan & Snidman, 2004; Kagan, Snidman, Kahn, & Towsley, 2007; Kagan, Snidman, McManis, Woodward, & Hardway, 2002). Carl Schwartz, who gathered fMRI data on these subjects at age 18, also found a shallower slope of habituation of the BOLD signal to the amygdala to unfamiliar events in the adolescents who had been high-reactive infants (Schwartz, Kunwar, Greve, Kagan, Snidman, & Bloch, 2012).

The temporal pattern of impulses arriving at a site can affect select outcomes. The temporal pattern in speech provides listeners with clues to the words that should be awarded emphasis when they infer the intended meaning. The sentence, "He went first to eat (pause) cookies" recruits attention to what was eaten, in this case cookies. The sentence, "He went first (pause) to eat cookies" recruits attention to the word *first* and implies that the agent ate more after partaking of the cookies.

The temporal pattern of inputs to the basolateral complex of the rat amygdala provides a persuasive illustration of the significance of this kind of incentive. The animals received two different patterns of six 10 msec bursts, interspersed with 10 msec intervals without electrical stimulation. Each pattern was used as a conditioned stimulus, with shock as the unconditioned stimulus and freezing as the conditioned response. Pattern A was 1001111001; pattern B was 1110000111 (1 represents a stimulus and 0 no stimulus). Although both patterns evoked conditioned freezing, pattern A was correlated with greater c-fos activity in the prefrontal cortex; pattern B with greater c-fos activity in the hypothalamus (Mourao, Lockmann, Castro, Medeiros, Reis, Pereira, et al., 2016).

Age, Class, Ethnicity, and Gender

A subject's age participates in a number of patterns that contribute to immune function, brain anatomy and function, and health because of maturation as well as variation in the life styles of older and younger members of the same family (He, Sillanpaa, Silventoinen, Kaprio, & Pitkaniemi, 2016; Silvers, Insel, Powers, Franz, Helion, Martin et al., 2016). Age accounted for more variation in brain morphology than the diseases of Parkinson's, schizophrenia, or autism (Sabuncu, Ge, Holmes, Smoller, Buckner, & Fischl, 2016). Although many investigators measure the cortical thickness of an entire lobe, the pattern of thickness in sulci and gyri differs in younger and older subjects. Only those younger than 14 years showed an inverse relation between sulcal and gyral thickness in frontal, temporal, and parietal sites

(Vandekar, Shinohara, Raznahan, Hopson, Roalf, Ruparel, et al., 2016). Age of onset of a symptom is often a clue to etiology. Adults who develop obsessive-compulsive symptoms in middle age differ from those who first displayed their symptoms in childhood (Sharan, Sundar, Thennarasu, & Reddy, 2015).

A person's social class during their childhood years is a consistent element in patterns that predict variation in cognitive abilities, academic achievement, personality, violent behavior, and physical and mental health across many societies. The reason for this robust fact is that membership in a class is associated with variation in prenatal health, parental practices, diet, medical care, quality of schooling, and opportunities for choice (Prins, Bates, Keyes, & Muntaner, 2015; Schiff, Duyme, Dumaret, Stewart, Tomkiewicz, & Feingold, 1978; Byrd, Hawes, Loeber, & Pardini, 2016; McLeod, Horwood, & Fergusson, 2016; Sariaslan, Larsson, & Fazel, 2016; Rentfrow, Jakela, & Lamb, 2015).

Class differences in language, especially size of vocabulary, appear as early as the second birthday (Kagan, Kearsley, & Zelazo, 1978). I worked in the small Mayan village of San Marcos la Laguna in northwest Guatemala, with a population of about 800 during the 1970s. Although every house was small, had a dirt floor, and no running water, the children from the small number of families who owned the tiny plot of land on which their house rested attained higher scores on the tests of cognitive talents we administered than those whose families rented the land.

Most children become aware of the signs of wealth or poverty by their fifth birthday and evaluate wealthy families as possessing more desirable traits (Shutts, Brey, Dornbusch, Slywotzky, & Olson, 2016). Youth from less advantaged families are continually exposed to the material goods, academic skills, and sense of agency of those who enjoy a more affluent childhood. A refusal to conform to the expectations of the majority is, for some, the only way to assert one's agency.

Lynsley Hanley, who grew up in a lower-middle-class family in England's West Midlands during the 1980s, captured the powerlessness and hunger for respectability among her peers (Hanley, 2016). The tension between al-Qaida and ISIS is partly due to a class difference in their recruits. The former draw mainly from better educated, professional groups, while ISIS receives many of its supporters from the lower middle class.

Class can exert its influence prenatally, as well as during the post-natal years. Brain scans of African-American infant girls born at term in a Philadelphia hospital revealed that the 25 percent of the sample born to the poorest, least educated women had less cortical gray matter than those born to more advantaged mothers (Betancourt, Avants, Farah, Brodsky, Wu, Ashtari, & Hurt, 2016), However, newborns possess considerable malleability. Children who begin life in poverty but manage to acquire 12 or more years of education are less susceptible to a depression or a cold following injection with a rhinovirus (Miller, Cohen, Janicki-Deverts, Brody, & Chen, 2016).

Individuals who had been diagnosed with ADHD as a child and also as an adult were more likely to have grown up in a disadvantaged family than those who received this diagnosis at only one age (Moffitt, Houts, Asherson, Belsky, Corcoran, Hammerle et al., 2015). The white, urban, American males between ages 18 and 25 who, in 2015, used opioid pain killers were at the highest risk for abusing heroin if they grew up in a family whose income was below the median (Compton, Jones, & Baldwin, 2016). Adults from disadvantaged backgrounds commit most of the acts of murder, forcible rape, or armed robbery in Sweden.

As a result, the heritability of these behaviors is low among this group because their life circumstances make a major contribution to these outcomes. The heritability of the same behaviors is higher among affluent Swedes for whom biological properties play a more important role (Frisell, Lichtenstein, & Langstrom, 2011). A child's social class can, under some circumstances, be as powerful a predictor of later criminal activity as parental abuse or neglect (Milaniak & Widom, 2015).

The previous chapter described the power of a person's identification with their family pedigree. Youth identify with their social class if it has distinctive features. American adolescents from poor families recognize the distinctiveness of their homes and neighborhoods. Those who identify with their class are likely to believe that they are susceptible to acquiring some of the undesirable traits they see in their friends and relatives, including poor grades, violence, and unemployment. Because the gap in income in the United States between the lowest and highest quintiles has increased over the past 40 years, a large, but unknown, proportion of poor Americans in 2016 are identified with their class.

The experiences associated with class membership can affect the genome. American adolescents who grew up in an advantaged family displayed a smaller increase in methylation of CpG islands in the promoter region of the serotonin transporter gene over a three-year interval than less advantaged youth (Swartz, Hariri, & Williamson, 2016). Yet, many investigators who discover a relation between a gene or epigenetic mark and a brain measure or illness ignore the participants' social class (Park, Lee, Kim, Cho, Yun, Han, et al., 2015; Duman & Canli, 2015; Muehlhan, Kirschbaum, Wittchen, & Alexander, 2015). The genes that are known risk factors for obesity and heart disease have a decreasing influence on the development of a health disability as a person's social class rises (Dinescu, Horn, Duncan, & Turkheimer, 2016). That is why a pattern that combines one or more risk alleles with the individual's social class is a better predictor of many outcomes than the alleles alone (Lahti, Raikkonen, Peltonen, Raitakari, & Keltikangas-Jarvinen, 2006; Nobile, Giorda, Marino, Carlet, Pastore, Vanzin, et al., 2007; Manuck, Flory, Ferrell, & Muldoon, 2004; Turkheimer, Haley, Waldron, D'Onofrio, & Gottesman, 2003).

Unfortunately, it is difficult to repair all the undesirable consequences of continued membership in a disadvantaged class. The government's Head Start program for young children was intended to reduce the seriousness of some of these consequences. Sadly, poor children, whether black, white, Asian, or Hispanic, who attended a Head Start program during the preschool years did not have better school-related skills at age five (vocabulary, letter identification) than those who did not receive the intervention. The reasons for this disappointing result are the substantial variation in the quality of the Head Start programs across the nation and the more profound influence of the home environment (Love, Chazan-Cohen, Raikes, & Brooks-Gunn, 2013).

Youth whose family pedigrees are marked by wealth and community respect for at least two generations are biased to assume that they are entitled to occupy positions of authority, Hence, they feel comfortable exercising the power that a position of authority requires. By contrast, many youths from family pedigrees marked by poverty and a compromised status for two or more generations hold a rebellious attitude toward high-status persons and resist awarding them any special virtue. A fair proportion of these adults feel less comfortable in a position of authority because they are reluctant to assume a role that they resented when they were adolescents. Youth who hold these ideas need someone to reassure them of their talents and legitimate right to an elite position.

Colin McGinn, a respected American philosopher who grew up in a working-class British family, wrote about the importance of the encouragement he received from a college professor. "It is hard to exaggerate the importance of this type of contact between students and teachers; for you to believe in yourself, someone else you respect has to believe in you first" (McGinn, 2002, p. 31). Bertrand Russell, who grew up in an elite family, would not have needed this source of support to believe in his intellectual abilities and his right to enjoy community respect.

Ethnicity is a third element in many patterns because the world's ethnic groups possess dissimilar genomes and, within a society, some groups hold distinct values (Zhu, Manichaikul, Hu, Chen, Liang, Steffen, et al., 2016). Hispanics were the only group in a large sample of older Americans that combined many stressful events during the prior two years, homozygosity for the short allele of the serotonin transporter gene, and increased risk for a bout of depression (Arpawong, Lee, Phillips, Crimmins, Levine, & Prescott, 2016). Although white and Hispanic preschool girls who participated in Tulsa's CAP Head Start program profited from the intervention, based on achievement test scores seven years later, African-American boys in the same program did not (Phillips, Gormley, & Anderson, 2016).

European-Caucasians and East Asians differ in patterns of alleles, experiences, and values that affect behavior, perception, and brain profiles (Han, Northoff, Vogeley, Wexler, Kitayana, & Varnum, 2013; Bodde 1991; Nisbett, Peng, Choi, & Norenzayan,

2001; Chua, Boland, & Nisbett, 2005; Pornpattananangkul, Hariri, Harada, Mano, Komeda, Parrish, et al., 2016; Immordino-Yang, Yang, & Damasio, 2014). Three-year-old Japanese children perform better than Americans on problems requiring holistic perception, for example detecting whether one object in a collection differs in orientation from others. But American toddlers do better than the Japanese on tasks requiring local processing, for example, inferring an object from a few of its features (Kuwabara & Smith, 2016).

The social scientists who hire volunteers from the Mechanical Turk website as subjects for studies seem unconcerned with the fact that a majority are well-educated, unemployed residents of India who are not religious and report higher than normative levels of social anxiety and depression (Paolacci & Chandler 2014; Arditte, Cek, Shaw, & Timpano, 2016). A similar criticism applies to studies that include only American college students (Henrich, Heine, & Norenzayan, 2010). Neither group is representative of any population.

Gender is a fourth component in patterns that predict personality, mental illness, physiology, brain anatomy and function, methylation patterns in fetal genomes, or select cognitive processes in humans and animals. Children recognize some of the obvious sex differences in behavior by the second birthday (Hill & Flom, 2007).

The varied effects of testosterone on the brain and body, prenatally as well as postnatally, are an important reason for the differences between males and females (Barth, Villringer, & Sacher, 2015; Tomasi & Volkow, 2012; Spiers, Hannon, Schalkwyk, Smith, Wong, O'Donovan, et al., 2015; Hamel, Lutz, Coleman, Worlein, Peterson, Rosenberg, et al., 2017; Vied, Ray, Badger, Bundy, Arbeitman, & Nowakowski, 2016). Male brains have greater connectivity within each hemisphere; whereas connectivity in female brains is greater between the two hemispheres (Ingalhalikar, Smith, Parker, Satterthwaite, Elliott, Ruparel et al., 2014).

The prenatal secretion of testosterone by male fetuses affects neurons in the parietal lobe that contribute to the solving of mental rotation problems and the perception of movement (Balconi & Cortesi 2015; Connolly, Kentridge, & Cavina-Pratesi, 2016). A small region within the visual cortex that is especially responsive to motion was larger in the right hemisphere of all five postmortem brains of older men but in only three of five female brains (Amunts, Armstrong, Malikovic, Homke, Mohlberg, Schleicher, & Zilles, 2007).

Although sex differences in average scores on most cognitive tasks are minimal, more males than females attain very high scores on tasks requiring mental manipulations of objects in space, a skill that is mediated in a major way by right parietal sites (Spetch & Parent, 2006; Koscik, O'Leary, Moser, Andreassen, & Nopoulos, 2009).

More boys than girls manipulate and draw objects that move, such as cars, balls, and trucks (Berenbaum & Beltz 2016; Turgeon, 2008; Iijima, Arisaka, Minamoto, & Arai, 2001). Young male monkeys and chimpanzees are also more likely than females to pick up objects that move when manipulated, such as leaves and sticks (Hassett, Siebert, & Wallen, 2008; Koops, Furuichi, Hashimoto, & van Schaik, 2015; Alexander & Hines 2002). Seven-month-old infants saw an adult punching or cradling a balloon. The infant boys looked longer at the former and were ikely to imitate that action when given the balloon. The girls, by contrast, looked longer at the cradling behavior and chose to imitate that response (Benenson, Tennyson, & Wrangham, 2011).

Can Statistics Detect Single Causes?

The social scientists who believe that some events possess a causal potency that does not require the addition of other conditions often rely on statistics to provide an estimate of the contribution of a single condition to an outcome. It is worth noting that biologists would not use these techniques to control for the contributions of average rainfall and soil quality in order to discover the contribution of temperature to the height of a rose plant because they appreciate that the effect of temperature on plant growth depends on the other two conditions. Roses do not grow in a warm region with sandy soil and no rain. The practice of using statistics to remove the contribution of sex to an outcome ignores the fact that males and females with similar mean values on all measures can display significantly different patterns of correlations.

Structural equation modeling (SEM), the most popular procedure for estimating the contribution of single events, requires four conditions that are not always met or even checked by investigators. The equations require linear relations among the variables, normative distributions without outliers, a ratio of 20 subjects for each parameter, and an a priori plan to examine a small number of relations. The first condition is the hardest to meet because nonlinear relations are common (Lahey, Lee, Sibley, Applegate, Molina, & Pelham, 2016). There is a nonlinear relation between the loudness of a sound and its discriminability, between the wavelength of electromagnetic radiation and its capacity to harm the body, and between annual income and subjective well-being. The attempts to control for the contribution of social class ignore the nonlinear relations between income or education, on the one hand, and incarceration, career choice, abuse of children, and the probability of dropping out of school. Rare or infrequent outcomes are also a problem. A sensitive predictor of an outcome whose frequency is less than 1 percent will correctly classify those who actualize the outcome, but will err by incorrectly classifying many more who do not. Suicide is an example of a rare outcome that is difficult to predict. The prevalence of suicide in the United States has averaged between 12 and 15 per 100,000 over the past century. There are about 250 million Americans over age 15 who have the ability to end their lives. The estimated 27,000 Americans who will kill themselves in 2016 are the outliers that Taleb (2007) calls black swans.

A majority of the statistically significant correlations social scientists report between two variables are attributable to the subjects whose values fell in the top or bottom 15 percent of the distribution. There is typically no relation for the remaining 70 percent of the sample. These relations are non-Gaussian; some are nonlinear. Salivary cortisol levels gathered from more than 18,000 persons of different ages in different laboratories during varied times of the day across the four seasons revealed that age, gender, laboratory, and season affected cortisol values. The occurrence of nonlinear relations between cortisol level and select outcomes implies the inappropriateness of relying on covariance statistics to control for age, gender, time of day, and season in an attempt to discover the contribution of cortisol to any outcome (Miller, Stalder, Jarczak, Almeida, Badrick, Bartels, et al. 2016).

The use of SEM can yield mischievous conclusions when the covariates are correlated with each other and/or with the outcome. When a covariance analysis removed the contributions of several indexes of a nation's economy in order to predict national suicide rates across 191 countries, the result implied that the nations with the largest numbers of psychiatrists had the highest suicide rates (Rajkumar, Brinda, Duba, Thangadurai, & Jacob, 2013). Investigators who controlled for the contribution of an informant's income, level of education, and employment (which are correlated) in order to estimate the contribution of a person's state of residence to judgments of subjective well-being found that Louisiana residents are the most satisfied Americans (Oswald & Wu, 2010). This so-called fact rubs against the more substantial observation that more Americans move to California than to Louisiana.

The counterintuitive conclusions that often emerge from such analyses are one reason why Nisbett (2015), Kraemer (2015), Wheelan (2013), and Infurna and Luthar (2016) are critical of the permissive and often inappropriate use of SEM and other covariance techniques. John Tukey (1969), who enjoyed the respect of all statisticians, warned investigators about the dangers of bending their question to fit a popular statistical procedure. This practice may yield a statistically significant result, but most significant findings have little theoretical importance. I often applied a covariance analysis to a set of data I had already examined in great detail in order to see whether its results corresponded to the inferences I had arrived at initially. In many instances the outcomes of the covariance analyses did not capture, and occasionally distorted, the relations that were present in the raw data.

Enrico Fermi appreciated the importance of understanding a phenomenon before applying fancy mathematics. When, in 1953, Freeman Dyson brought Fermi a set of theoretical calculations pertaining to scattering experiments the older physicist told Dyson, "There are two ways of doing calculations in theoretical physics. One way, and this is the way I prefer, is to have a clear physical picture of the process you are calculating. The other way is to have a precise and self-consistent mathematical formalism. You have neither" (Segre & Hoerlin, 2016, p. 273). Fermi would have been unhappy with the widespread practice of using covariance statistics to illuminate phenomena that are incompletely understood, such as subjective well-being or depression,

Persons Not Variables

The significance of patterns is one reason why Bergman (1998) has urged scientists studying psychological outcomes in humans to replace the current focus on relations among continuous variables across persons with classes of individuals defined by their pattern of features. The challenge of predicting which young scientists are most likely to make a major discovery requires knowledge of their personal properties, as well as their past and present life circumstances. That is why the timing of the most influential research of scientists from one of seven disciplines was randomly distributed within a particular investigator's total body of work (Sinatra, Wang, Deville, Song, & Barabasi, 2016).

The career of Ernest O. Lawrence, who invented the cyclotron, is illustrative. Lawrence had to possess special intellectual abilities, unlimited energy, and vaulting ambition. But this trio of personal properties had to be combined with at least three other events that were beyond his control. The president of the University of California during the 1920s had to be so eager to establish a first-class university with an impressive physics department that he was willing to give the 28-year-old Lawrence money and space that no other president would have offered a young, unknown scientist. In addition, bright graduate students had to select the physics department at Berkeley, rather than Princeton, Harvard, or Yale, as the place to study, and senior physicists had to be receptive to new ways to study the nucleus of the atom (Hiltzik, 2015).

The patterns of BOLD signals in 14 adults solving varied memory tasks, measured on two occasions separated by two months, implied that each person had a stable and unique pattern that was hidden when average BOLD values were computed across all subjects (Miller, Donovan, Van Horn, German, Sokol-Hessner, & Wolford, 2009). The same result was found for resting-state functional connectivity patterns in adults scanned on multiple occasions. The connectivity pattern was more reliable within than across subjects (Langs, Wang, Golland, Mueller, Pan, Sabancu, et al., 2016; Shine, Koyejo, & Poldrack, 2016).

Latent class analysis is well suited to discovering types of persons (Lanza & Cooper, 2016). This method yields categories analogous to the biological concept of species. Many children who are unusually bold in unfamiliar settings possess greater GABAergic activity in the basomedial nucleus of the amygdala, a Caucasian pedigree, dark eyes and hair, a mesomorphic body build, and a broad face (Kagan, 1994; Mesquita, Abreu, de Abreu, de Souza, de Noronha, Silva, et al., 2016). By contrast, a pattern defined by blue eyes, blond hair, an ectomorphic body build, a narrow face, and a low threshold for detecting the smell of butanol in water is more characteristic of shy, male college students (Herbener, Kagan, & Cohen, 1989).

Most papers reporting the average magnitudes of a brain measure, across subjects, fail to tell readers the proportion of subjects who displayed large, moderate, or negligible changes and the properties of those in each group. A study of the blood levels of 13 different cytokines in a sample of 262 healthy, adolescent

American girls containing 62 percent white and 32 percent black youths points to the value of examining the proportion of subjects in varied groups. A factor analysis of the measures across subjects yielded four factors representing variation in innate or adaptive immunity. However, this analysis did not tell readers that only seven percent of the group had high concentrations of all the cytokines and this group had more black than white girls (Dorn, Gayles, Engelwood, Houts, Cizza, & Denson, 2016).

The percentage of the American population in each of six income brackets adds information about the nation's economic health that is more informative than mean income level. Government officials regularly publish the proportion of Americans in different age and ethnic groups who were burdened with each major disease during the previous year. This information tells us more than the mean number of visits to a physician or the average number of days in a hospital across diseases, ages, and class or ethnic groups.

The absence of words that describe kinds of individuals contributes to the resistance to adopting this strategy. The popularity of concepts defined by continuous measures, such as extraversion, coping ability, and effortful control, sustains the reliance on analyses of variance and correlations computed on continuous measures across subjects. It is not uncommon, however, for a group of subjects to have similar mean values on four measures and belong to one of three groups possessing different patterns of values on the measures (Gates & Molenaar, 2012). It is this fact that lends support to the validity of Bergman's advice.

It is easier to compute the correlation between being a victim of bullying and later measures of anxiety or depression, controlling for correlated variables with covariance techniques, than to combine victimhood, a disadvantaged social class, ethnicity, academic problems, and gender into a single predictor for which no name exists. The practice of treating the extraversion scale on the Big Five questionnaire as having the same meaning in recidivist male criminals who grew up in disadvantaged families, female politicians who enjoyed affluent childhoods, and college students from different ethnic and social class groups is not leading to important insights.

Biologists do not compute the average height of plants from four genetic strains growing at one of four altitudes because they know that the height of each strain is a product of a unique pattern of genes and altitude that is not predictable from either genes or altitude alone. Humans and chimpanzees share more than 98 percent of the same genes, but these genes assume distinctive patterns in the two species. A biologist would not perform an analysis of variance on a measure of "ability to cope with frustration" on samples that combined Pan and bonobo chimpanzees, orangutans, gorillas, and gibbons because this trait is only one element in patterns that differentiate the five ape species (Vinken, Van den Bergh, Vermaercke, & Op de Beeck, 2016).

The study of infant temperamental biases in different ethnic groups affirms the wisdom of searching for kinds of individuals. The mean values on limb activity, crying, and salivary cortisol were similar in four-month-old European- and Chinese-American infant boys and girls exposed to unexpected visual and auditory events. However, the patterns these three variables assumed were different among the four ethnicity by gender groups. Only among Caucasian males was there a group that combined high levels of motor activity and frequent crying with high baseline levels of cortisol (Liu, Snidman, & Kagan, 2016, unpublished).

Only 2 of 46 infant boys classified as low reactive at four months (defined by minimal motor activity and little crying to unexpected events) combined unusually low baseline heart rates with frequent smiling, minimal crying, and a fearless approach to unfamiliar objects and people during the second year (Kagan, Snidman, McManis, Woodward, & Hardway, 2002). As an adolescent, one of these boys forged his parents' signature on a letter that he mailed to the admissions committee of a private school which declined acceptance to the school. The second boy, at age 15, told an interviewer who had asked about his adult vocational plans that he was considering running for president of the United States. These two boys possess a rare pattern of traits that had its origins in a special blend of genes and experiences. The answers to the Big Five questionnaire provided by a large sample of adolescents that included these two boys would not reveal their unusual personality.

The evidence invites a change in current research strategies. Investigators should examine relations between patterns of causal conditions and outcome measures. It is time for scientists studying psychological outcomes to acknowledge the rarity of silver bullet causes and to accept the complexity hiding in every computer printout.

6 Attributing Psychological Properties to Brain Profiles

The constraint on the validity of inferences based on one source of evidence bears directly on the neuroscientist's habit of describing brain profiles with words whose meaning and validity originated in psychological data. This practice deserves careful scrutiny because animals or humans are the presumed agents in sentences containing terms describing the psychological processes of perception, memory, intention, feeling, emotion, reasoning, or action. These terms take on novel meanings in sentences in which neuronal activity is the noun (Searle, 2003).

English-speaking four-year-olds accept the legitimacy of sentences in which an inanimate object is the cause of an event, as in "The microwave heated the coffee." Japanese four-year-olds accept only an animate agent as the noun in sentences implying a causal influence on a target (Kanero, Hirsh-Pasek, & Golinkoff, 2016). Presumably, if Japanese children understood what neurons did, they would reject sentences in which neurons caused a psychological outcome.

The practice of using psychological predicates, such as compute, regulate, or synthesize, to describe brain profiles remains popular because neuroscientists do not have a rich biological vocabulary for the diverse brain profiles that occur in response to incentives. The terms "resting default state" and "coherence of oscillation frequencies between sites" are exceptions, but many more concepts are needed. Molecular biologists do not borrow the words that describe the properties of proteins and apply them to the nucleotide sequences that are their foundations. Neither do physicists apply the concepts appropriate for molecules to quantum particles. Every observable phenomenon consists of a cascade of phases. The entities and functions of each phase require their own vocabulary.

Gyorgy Buzsaki (2016) is also troubled by the habit of labeling brain profiles with terms for mental states. Brain states consist of continually changing patterns of voltages, frequencies, and molecular deformations in varying numbers of neurons at distinctive locations for varying durations. Although these states are the foundation of all psychological phenomena, it is impossible at the moment to explain how the latter emerge from the former. The choice of the phrase "top-down control" to describe the effects on recall memory that are the result of connections between the prefrontal cortex and the entorhinal region and hippocampus was unfortunate because it evokes the image of an executive giving orders to subordinates.

The short life of many psychological concepts makes it unlikely that a majority of contemporary terms will map neatly on brain profiles. If magnetic scanners had been available in Ivan Pavlov's laboratory in 1900 he might have assigned the freedom reflex to a brain site. Advocates of Freudian ideas might have been tempted to attribute the processes that define the oral stage, id, and superego to brain profiles. Sigmund Freud once drew a sketch in which he placed the id in posterior brain regions, the ego in the prefrontal cortex, and the superego in the temporal lobe.

The popular concept of reward has an important origin in Thorndike's positing of the Law of Effect (Thorndike, 1898). Thorndike, like others of his generation, was influenced by the late-nineteenth-century American pragmatists Charles Peirce, William James, and Chauncey Wright. These scholars favored functional definitions of concepts whose features had an observable effect on the world, rather than definitions that specified intrinsic properties. Later generations reified this term by treating it as a natural kind with a location in the brain.

Communities invent words to serve a pragmatic need. Many common phenomena lack a semantic name in most languages. There is no English word for the lowest branch on a tree or the largest puddle on a trail, even though these features are occasionally noticed. Moreover, superordinate terms, which are frequent in psychology, are usually invented after their concrete exemplars are named (Brown, 1958). The first humans wanted to know where a fig or deer could be found, not where food or an animal was located.

Psychologists are attracted to superordinate concepts, while the public prefers the concrete exemplars. Psychologists use the term *aggression* to name any member of a diverse collection of acts that harm another or appear to threaten harm. The public prefers words like *hit*, *stab*, *shoot*, *rob*, *push*, or *insult*. Psychologists choose the word *stress* to name experiences as varied as unemployment, poverty, illness, loss of a friend, overwork, or death of a parent. Superordinate terms require other words to disambiguate their meaning (Earles & Kersten, 2016),. The meanings of *slap* and *unemployed* are less ambiguous than *aggression* and *stress*. German adults reading nouns and verbs that referred to concrete events showed increased activity in the corrugator muscle of the forehead to words such as *vomit* and *strangle*, but not to the superordinate terms *illness* and *aggression* (Kunecke, Sommer, Schacht, & Palazova, 2015).

Natural scientists are skeptical of the validity of statements that originate in intuition. It is surprising, therefore, that neuroscientists are expending extraordinary effort looking for brain patterns that correspond to the intuitions that rationality, social impact, valence, and self are theoretically significant natural kinds that have specific locations in the brain (Tamir, Thornton, Contreras, & Mitchell, 2016; Babo-Rebelo, Richter, & Tallon-Baudry, 2016).

The abstract term *valence*, which refers to different kinds of sensations, events, people, objects, and actions, conflates quality of sensory feeling with value judgments of actions and people. Neurons in the basolateral amygdala are activated by odors that animals avoid. These neurons are responding to inputs from olfactory cortex generated by the features of the molecules comprising the odors (Jin, Zelano, Gottfried, & Mohanty, 2015; Namburi, Al-Hasani, Calhoon, Bruchas, & Tye, 2016).

Some neuroscientists contend that the brain can predict, chunk, recognize patterns, and detect meaning in recursive sentences (Dehaene, Meyniel, Wacongne, Wang, and Pallier, 2015). The meanings of these four concepts, and the validities of conclusions that rely on these concepts, originate in psychological evidence, usually gathered on conscious human subjects. After surveying the terms that many investigators used to describe BOLD signals in the striatum, one team assigned the labels *executive functions, action value,* and *social and language functions* to each of three locations in this site, even though the theoretical utility of this trio of concepts is still being debated (Pauli, O'Reilly, Yarkoni, & Wager, 2016).

The discovery of distinctive BOLD signals in undergraduates with some knowledge of physics reading about the concepts of causal motion, energy flow, and periodicity led the investigators to conclude that the active sites were processing these abstract concepts (Mason & Just, 2016). One problem with this claim is that these sites are activated when adults perform tasks that have no relation to physics (Tylen, Philipsen, Roepstorff, & Fusaroli, 2016). It is likely that the schemata evoked by reading about the physical concepts, together with the effort needed to perform the task, explain the profile of activated sites. There is considerable overlap between the sites that are activated when adults think about physical ideas and when they solve working memory problems (Fischer, Mikhael, & Kanwisher, 2016).

The Concept of Number

A sizeable number of scientists have been persuaded that the brains of animals and humans are biologically prepared to register and represent the number of elements in an array, in contrast to responding to the total area covered by a collection of objects, their size and density, or the total amount of contour. Combinations of these physical properties necessarily vary with the number of objects. It is impossible to prove that an animal or human perceives the number of things in an array, independent of these features. The many species that can be trained to discriminate between arrays with differing numbers of objects are probably relying on these features (Raphael & Morgan, 2016; Beran & Parrish, 2016).

An important source of evidence sustaining the conviction that the brain registers number is activity in the intraparietal sulcus (IPS) when humans or animals are discriminating between arrays containing different numbers of objects, usually black or white dots (Dehaene, 1997). However, there was little increase in activation of the intraparietal sulcus when students had to detect, in half-second exposures, changes in the number of shapes or the number of protrusions from a shape when the number was less than four. There was a large increase in the BOLD signal to the IPS when the number of shapes or protrusions was greater than four, probably because it was difficult to detect a change in such a brief exposure (Porter, 2016). Crows, who lack an IPS, can be trained to respond to arrays varying in number of dots. After training, individual neurons in a posterior site in the crow brain responded to an array with a particular number of dots (Ditz & Nieder, 2016). Because no neuron reacted to arrays containing varying numbers of dots, it is possible that the training tuned each cell to respond to a particular spatial pattern of closed contours.

The advocates promoting the view that the IPS registers number rarely cite the fact that two arrays of three objects evoked dissimilar BOLD patterns in the human IPS when the objects were equally spaced in one array, but in the other the two proximal objects were separated from the third. This result implies that the brain was responding to the spatial distribution of the objects rather than their number (Xu & Chun, 2007). Infants, too, are sensitive to changes in the spatial locations of objects. They display increased attention when, following familiarization on one spatial array of three objects, the locations of one or more objects were altered (Wiener & Kagan, 1976; Richmond, Zhao, & Burns, 2015).

The primary functions of the superior and inferior parietal lobules, which border the IPS and affect its activity, are to mediate saccades, activate schemata, guide accurate reaching, maintain attention, and detect the salient features in a sequence (Steenrod, Phillips, & Goldberg, 2013; Husain & Nachev, 2007; Caminiti, Chafee, Battaglia-Mayer, Averbach, Crowe, & Georgopoulos, 2010; Connolly, Kentridge, & Cavina-Pratesi, 2016; Madore, Szpunar, Addis, & Schacter, 2016;Ibos & Freedman, 2016; Shibata, Sasaki, Kawato, & Watanabe, 2016; Tudusciuc & Neider, 2009).

It is relevant that the profiles of BOLD signals to arrays of dots often differ from those evoked by Arabic numerals that correspond to the number of dots (Harvey, Klein, Petridou, & Dumoulin, 2013), although this is not always the case (Kadosh, Bahrami, Walsh, Butterworth, Popescu, & Price, 2011). School-age children subtracting two Arabic numbers showed a brain profile that differed from the one recorded when they subtracted arrays of black dots (Peters, Polspoel, Op de Beeck, & De Smedt, 2016; Bulthe, De Smedt, & Op de Beeck, 2015). This observation is inconsistent with the premise that the brain is especially tuned to register numerosity. Neither five-year-olds nor adults selected number as the best match of a target to one of four pictures when shape or color were alternatives (Chen & Mazzocco, 2017). These observations confirm the fact that humans rarely rely on number as the salient feature in scenes containing objects that vary in shape, size, color, motion, or function because it is usually the least informative feature. Few adults sitting in front of a plate containing a fork, knife, piece of fish, and potato would note that there were four objects on the plate.

The blood flow changes (recorded with near-infrared spectroscopy, or NIRS) in six-month-old infants exposed to sequences of 8 or 16 dots for one-second durations were restricted to the right parietal cortex. Because this site could not "count" the number of dots in such a brief interval, a reasonable inference is that the neurons were registering the spatial distribution of the dots (Edwards, Wagner, Simon, & Hyde, 2016).

There is, in addition, a weak predictive relation between an infant's ability to discriminate among arrays of dots and later mathematical achievement (LeFevre, 2016). Many five-year-olds who can count to ten do not understand that each number represents a distinct magnitude that increases across the sequence of names (Siegler, 2016). The collection of evidence led Cantrell & Smith (2013), Leibovich & Henik (2014), and Mix, Levine, & Newcombe (2016) to question the notion that infants who discriminate between arrays of dots, based on changes in total looking time or brain profiles, are responding primarily to the number of objects in the array. They argue, instead, that the infants, and by inference their brains, are detecting changes in the area covered by the array, the locations, size, or density of the objects, and/or the total amount of contour.

It is difficult to defend the hypothesis that the intraparietal sulcus in humans, monkeys, or homologous regions in birds, rats, or fish, all of which can be trained to discriminate between arrays that vary in number of objects, evolved to register the exact number of things in the visual field. It is adaptive to detect the difference between many pieces of food, predators, or mating partners and a few, but it is less obvious that the ability to perceive the exact number of these objects would aid fitness. It is more reasonable to presume that the spatial contiguity of the anterior section of the primate intraparietal sulcus, which mediates reaching for an object, and the lateral and posterior regions, which mediate detection of the spatial location of objects, implies that the primary function of the IPS is to locate objects in the visual field so that the organism will be able to seize, grab, or bite them (Zlatkina & Petrides, 2014).

The ability to distinguish between events that differ in their physical features does not imply an understanding of the abstract concepts that psychologists often impose on the stimulus or the evidence (Eger, 2016; Kagan, 2008; Haith, 1998; Cantrell & Smith, 2013). Infants display an increase in attention to lines that intersect after familiarization on a pair of parallel lines without any appreciation of the concept of parallel lines. Although infants could discriminate between a clock face that, in one picture, had one hand pointing to the 12 position and the other to the 6 and in a second picture had the hands pointing to 9 or 3, no one would claim that this perceptual talent meant that the infants understood anything about time. Pigeons can be trained to discriminate between letter sequences representing meaningful compared with meaningless words without any understanding of the semantic meanings of the words (Scarf, Boy, Reinart, Devine, Gunturkun, & Colombo, 2016).

The brain of a bee foraging from the hive to a food source registers the optic flow created by the contoured objects the bee flies over. This variable is usually correlated with distance from the hive. The changes in the brain generated by the optic flow determine the duration of the waggles the bee performs on the straight segment of the figure eight dance performed on returning to the hive (Shafir & Barron, 2010). The bee's brain does not register a number representing the distance from hive to food source. Psychologists prefer to use abstract terms to label observations that are more reasonably understood as consequences of the physical features of the events.

Animals perceive objects in different locations and event sequences with different delays. Our species invented symbolic concepts to represent the exact number of things, the distances between them, and the duration between events. A woman standing in a meadow facing one of its only two trees, which are 200 yards apart, could answer "one" or "two" if her friend asked, "How many trees do you see?" The correct reply depends on the extent of the visual field the woman assumed the friend had in mind when she asked the question. The numbers that specify quantity, distance, and time are not inherent in the physical events. Every known language invented words for one or two objects. Only a small number extended the vocabulary to cover any quantity of objects and the superordinate concept *number*. The mathematical concept of *set* is a relatively recent idea. That is why members of some Middle East societies 6000 years ago used different kinds of tokens to designate the same number of objects belonging to different categories, say 12 sheep versus 12 goats (Schmandt-Besserat, 1996). The speakers of most languages looking at a pig, a man, a rake, a log, and a bucket inside a wooden enclosure would not say that they saw five objects.

Concepts of Place and Time

The meanings and validities of statements claiming that neurons in the hippocampus encode space and time are not those humans understand when they think about the locations of familiar objects or the time elapsed between two events (Hasselmo & Stern, 2015; Howard & Eichenbaum, 2015). Mice and rats learn about their environment by moving through it. Hence, brain activity associated with the speed of limb movements, head orientation, and the presence of boundaries contribute to the brain's response in a location.

Neuroscientists write that place cells in the hippocampus represent the specific locations an animal encountered while running in a maze or on a rectangular or circular track. Howard Eichenbaum, the editor of the journal *Hippocampus*, commented that this phrasing is not quite correct. "The key factor is not differences in stimulus patterns associated with different directions, but rather whether the movement directions are meaningfully different (e.g., running in versus out of maze arms, following a path to obtain a series of food pellets). … The use of the term *place cell* … should not be interpreted [as meaning] that the cell actually measures place" (personal communication, 2016). The famous research subject H.M. navigated his environment successfully despite the loss of his hippocampus.

The neurons in the rat hippocampus labeled time cells are only active when the animal is engaged in a task, such as running in a wheel or inhibiting a response during a delay interval (Salz, Tiganj, Khasnabish, Kohley, Sheean, Howard, & Eichenbaum, 2016). It remains possible that this neuronal activity reflects feedback from muscles, vestibular neurons, and autonomic targets. Some of this information is relayed to the hippocampus through septal nuclei that are reciprocally connected with the medial entorhinal cortex (Tai & Leung, 2012). Each time an animal moves or changes the angle of its head, the resulting vestibular activity alters septal neurons whose projections contribute to the theta oscillations recorded in entorhinal and hippocampal sites (Gonzalez-Sulser, Parthier, Candela, McClure, Pastoll, Garden, et al., 2014).

Eichenbaum (personal communication, 2016) notes, "Time cells can be responding to an accumulation of vestibular activity on each run, or an accumulation of footsteps taken. … Both time and place cells reflect the associative organization of stimuli and events that are linked in time and/or space, and should not be thought of as cells that are driven by time or space per se. …

[The activity of these cells] is [only] correlated with the passage of time."

Every sequence is necessarily correlated with the passage of time. Telomere lengths shorten with the passage of time, but geneticists do not write that the DNA sequences of the telomeres are "time nucleotides." Neurons cannot code temporal intervals that transcend the context in which the interval occurs (Genovesio, Seitz, Tsujimoto, & Wise, 2016). Time can refer to the interval between two different events, different states of the same event, the changing positions of the hands on a clock, a person's subjective sense of the duration of an interval, or the meaning of space-time in Einstein's General Relativity equations (Jaroszkieicz, 2016). None of these meanings is identical with the meaning of the activity in the neurons called time cells.

Rather than use the words *place* and *time* to describe the activity of hippocampal neurons, it seems more accurate to write that a major function of the hippocampus is to bind all reward relevant stimuli into a representation that reflects the strengths of the associations among them (Eichenbaum, 2017). Every network of associations is acquired in particular locations at particular times.

The concept of consciousness provides a final example of a popular word that is unlikely to be instantiated in a particular pattern of neuronal activity (Popper & Eccles, 1977). Consciousness can refer to the awareness of an event or bodily state, the directing or altering of one's thoughts, or the feeling that the self is a unity (Feinberg & Mallatt, 2016). A person who has just awakened after a long night's sleep, is thinking about an uncomfortable meeting later in the day, or reflecting on her life history experiences three different states of consciousness. Although the subjective feeling and brain profile are likely to be different in each of the above states, English, but not all languages, invented a single word for these diverse phenomena. This semantic convention tempted some distinguished scientists to write about the neural correlates of consciousness as if the term named a single state that varied only in degree (Koch, Massimini, Boly, & Tononi, 2016; Bayne, Hohwy, & Owen, 2016).

The variation in select brain measures during the stages of sleep supports the notion of multiple forms of consciousness. There is an increase in low-frequency delta power and in the predictability of EEG features when humans move from being awake through the successive stages of light non-REM sleep, deep non-REM, and REM (rapid eye movement) sleep. The brain features in REM sleep imply a qualitatively distinct stage. Sleeping adults who were instructed to make a hand response upon hearing each of two categories of unfamiliar words showed a distinctive EEG waveform in light non-REM sleep, implying that their brains registered the words, but did not do so in REM sleep. However, the brain did display the distinctive waveform in REM sleep to words that were familiar because the subjects had seen them when awake (Andrillon, Poulsen, Hansen, Leger, & Kouider, 2016). This evidence favors the notion of qualitatively distinct forms of consciousness, rather than one state varying only quantitatively.

Are Words for Human Processes Appropriate for Animals?

The practice of assigning to animals psychological terms for processes that are likely to be restricted to human agents is burdened with the same problems that trail the use of these words to label brain states. One team studying olive flounder in a tank classified some fish as shy because they swam less than most fish and became immobile when a human attempted to capture them (Rupia, Binning, Roche, & Lu, 2016). The referents for shyness in a child or adult are a reluctance to talk, approach, or interact with strangers.

Other investigators thought it appropriate to use the word "egalitarian" to describe pairs of dogs in which neither animal was dominant (Trisko, Sandel, & Smuts, 2016), "anxious" to label avoidant behavior in crayfish, "intelligence" to describe select actions in parrots or monkeys, or a "sense of justice" to birds (Olkowicz, Kocourek, Lucan, Portes, Fitch, Herculano-Houzel, & Nemec, 2016; Fossat, Bacque-Cazenave, De Deurwaerdere, Delbecque, & Cattaert, 2014; Piantadosi & Kidd, 2016; Lents, 2016). I confess to surprise upon reading a paper that attributed the social anthropologist's concept of polyandry, which presumes a ritual of marriage, to the females of an invertebrate species who mated with many males (Michalczyk, Millard, Martin, Lumley, Emerson, Chapman, & Gage, 2011).

Nature is replete with examples of a species possessing a trait that is absent in other forms. Bats use the echo of sounds they emit from their mouth to detect a moving insect; penguin fathers tend the egg they fertilized through a long winter; bonobos engage in sex when distressed. Our species also possesses a number of unique psychological processes (Penn, Holyoak, & Povenelli, 2008). They include the ability to infer others' feelings and thoughts as well as hypothetical events, an understanding of right and wrong, the classification of outcomes as fair or unfair, a capacity for empathy, guilt, and shame, identifications with persons and groups, a desire to affirm self's virtue and dignity, a symbolic language with a recursive syntax, and a conscious awareness of self as a sensing agent who is responsible for his or her behaviors. No other animal possesses this collection of properties. That is one reason why mice have been a poor guide to understanding mental illnesses and developing effective drug therapies for the symptoms (Hyman, 2016).

An appreciation of right and wrong actions emerges in all children before the third birthday, and from that time forward every human with an intact brain spends the hours when they are not tending to bodily needs trying to obtain or maintain assurance that they are worthy of affection and respect. No primatologist has observed a vocal call or gesture in an ape that resembled a reprimand or saw a chimpanzee share some of his food with another because he felt he received more than he deserved (Ulber, Hamann, & Tomasello, 2016). It is difficult to imagine an ape wondering why the sun disappears at the end of each day or experiencing auditory hallucinations accusing the animal of a sin and ordering an act of self-harm (McCarthy-Jones, 2012).

This collection of unique human traits was made possible by patterns of anatomical and physiological features that are unique to the human brain (Nunez & Srinivasan, 2007; Aldridge, 2011). For example, the von Economo neurons in fronto-polar regions of human brains have morphological features that are missing from ape brains (Stimpson, Tetreault, Allman, Jacobs, Butti, Hof, & Sherwood, 2011). In addition, analyses of cholinergic and dopaminergic innervation of the basal ganglia in postmortem chimpanzee, gorilla, and human brains revealed that humans, compared with both ape species, had much less cholinergic innervation of sections of the caudate nucleus and more dopaminergic than cholinergic innervation of most of the striatum (Stephenson, Edler, Erwin, Jacobs, Hopkins, Hof, Sherwood, & Roshanti, 2017). This neurochemical pattern would allow humans to avoid states of hyper-vigilance and the inflexible repetition of stereotyped responses.

Many animal behaviors that resemble human actions in surface features originate in different causal conditions (Hecht, Murphy, Gutman, Votaw, Schuster, Preuss, et al., 2013). Actions that harm another provide an example. A male zebra fish often bites another while defending a territory or competing for a resource. Male fruit flies competing for a female spread their wings, lunge, and butt heads with a rival. Some rhesus monkeys shake their cage when an unfamiliar human stares at them. Investigators see no problem in calling these acts examples of aggression (Chou, Amo, Kinoshita, Cherng, Shimazaki, Agetsuma et al., 2016; Penn, Zito, & Kravitz, 2010; Hamel, Lutz, Coleman, Worlein, Peterson, Rosenberg, et al., 2017). Aggressive behaviors in humans, however, require the agent to have an intention to harm a victim (Ames & Fiske, 2013). The brain profiles that mediate intentional acts of slapping, stabbing, shooting, spitting, robbing, gossiping, rejecting, or torturing another person are unlikely to resemble the brain states that mediate biting in zebra fish or shaking one's cage in monkeys. Most human aggression is the product of inconsistencies in the networks that define self's virtue and potency. That is why labeling a zebra fish that bites another animal as "aggressive" represents a a serious change in the meaning of the term. Some investigators are sensitive to this issue. Scheel, Godfrey-Smith, and Lawrence (2016) used the term "grappling" to describe the behavior of an octopus that displayed a raised mantle when interacting with another displaying the same feature.

A second-by-second analysis of a cat's behavior with a mouse revealed a sequence that began with the cat swiping a paw at the mouse, followed by mouth contact, and finally biting. The latter act appeared to be the inevitable outcome of the increase in arousal that accompanied continued interaction with the mouse (Pellis, O'Brien, Pellis, Teitelbaum, Wolgin, & Kennedy, 1988). The fact that the mouse was eventually killed does not warrant calling the cat's behavior "aggressive," because there is no evidence to suggest that the cat intended to kill the mouse when the sequence began. The lion that attacks a gazelle and the crocodile that snaps at a fish do not have a conscious intention to harm these targets. They are simply hungry.

Equally important, some human behaviors that do harm another are not examples of aggression. Nursing infants who bite their mother's nipple do not intend to hurt the parent. A person carrying a dangerous microbe who unwittingly infects a friend did not intend to do harm. The ability to infer the thoughts or feelings of another, which is a critical feature in intentions to harm another, appears in most children by the second birthday. Infants as young as 18 months infer that a person pointing at an object is communicating a desire for the object. Orangutans, which are closer relatives of humans than zebra fish, who see someone pointing at a box containing food fail to infer that the person wants the food (Moore, Call, & Tomasello, 2015). Two-year-olds who had worn opaque ski goggles at home for an hour a day over several days returned to a laboratory room where their mother put on the ski goggles. These children became puzzled when the parent asked her son or daughter to bring her a particular toy because their past experience led them to infer that the goggles must have imposed the same state of blindness on the mother as they did on them (Kagan, 1981).

A fair proportion of two-year-old children from diverse cultures cried when an adult, who had just acted out several difficult actions with toys, said, "Now it's your turn to play." They

became distressed because they inferred that the adult expected
then to perform the same tasks and they sensed their inability
to do so (Kagan, 1981). No young chimp would become upset
if an adult animal who had seized some fruit from a branch
high on a tree signaled to the juvenile to do the same. Most
young children watching an examiner hide a toy in the top,
middle, or bottom tier of one box infer that the prize is located
in the corresponding tier of an adjacent box. Orangutans cannot solve this problem and chimpanzees do not perform as well
as children (Christie, Gentner, Call, Benjamin, & Haun, 2016).
Chimpanzees have great difficulty learning that if they point
to the smaller amount of food they will receive a larger por-
tion (Beran, James, Withan, & Parrish, 2016). Children solve
this problem in a few trials because they detect similarities in
the relations between events, such as the smaller of two objects,
that are not limited to specific settings. An early study reporting that chimpanzees explore the location of a mirror reflection
of a mark on their body claimed that this evidence meant that
apes possessed a representation of self. Later work revealed that
only a minority of apes display this behavior; whereas almost
all three-year-olds will touch their nose when they see a red
mark on this site while looking at a mirror (Hecht, Mahovetz,
Preuss, & Hopkins, 2016).

I suspect that one of the rationales for using terms naming
human properties to describe animal behaviors, aggression is an
example, rests on the premise that if animals and humans see,
smell, hear, eat, move, and breathe, it is reasonable to expand
the set of similarities to other properties. This is an example of
the logical argument called the error of the consequent, which
assumes the following form: If A then B; B; therefore A. This fal-
lacy is clear when applied to infants. Infants see, smell, eat, hear,

move, and breathe, but are incapable of an intention to harm someone.

No one denies that apes and humans share similar biological bases for many processes, including perception, short term memory, locomotion, hunger, and thirst. But that fact does not imply the real possibility that some human capacities are restricted to our species. Bacteria and yeast share many biological features, but the presence of a nucleus in yeast renders it qualitatively different from all prokaryotes. The appearance of a notochord, lung, internal fertilization, and convoluted cortex were equally distinctive evolutionary novelties. That is why it is not blasphemous to argue that a number of human psychological functions are missing from the repertoire of apes.

It is easy to cherry-pick a species possessing a trait that resembles a human property and conclude that this species, and perhaps others as well, possesses a form of the trait. Gibbons bond to a mate, but chimpanzees are sexually promiscuous. Baboons are sociable, but orangutans are solitary. Rhesus macaque mothers care for their infants but among titi monkeys it is the fathers who are the primary caretakers. Male elephant seals dominate harems of females, but among elephants it is the females that are dominant. Nature has enough diversity to defend almost any statement about psychological similarities between animals and humans.

The media contribute to the belief that animals share a number of traits with humans by reporting that crows, parrots, or chimpanzees possess a competence that had been thought to be restricted to humans. One rarely reads about the discovery of an ability that was uniquely human. There are several reasons for this asymmetry in reporting.

First, the articles and television programs describing the increasing rates of extinction of many species have generated public concern for these victims of human behavior. Any evidence that renders them more human should aid conservation efforts. It is also relevant that many contemporary adults regard our species as selfish, aggressive, and destructive, in contrast to the eighteenth century's gentler view of *Homo sapiens* as thoughtful, creative, and rational. This dark image of our species makes it easy to perceive similarities between a lion killing a gazelle and a youth shooting a peer. Many who are unhappy with the malevolent image of our species hope to alter this evaluation by advocating a kinder treatment of animals. This mission would be easier to promote if the scientific evidence pointed to basic similarities between animals and us.

Finally, the premise of a smooth, continuous gradation between animals and humans rationalizes research on animals that is designed to find the causes of psychiatric disorders such as autism, schizophrenia, depression, or social anxiety. It remains possible, however, that only humans can suffer from these disorders. Although animals and humans share genes that render some humans susceptible to the biology that contributes to one of these disorders, the defining symptoms often require either language impairment, illogical thought sequences, guilt, or shame. These phenomena are unique to our species.

The scientists who believe in a seamless continuity of psychological capacities between apes and humans do not seem to appreciate that this premise implies that the genes responsible for the unique physical properties of the human brain and body make no contribution to the special qualities of human inference, memory, emotion, language, and reasoning. This division between the physical and the mental is unlikely. For example, the flatter facial skeleton of humans, compared with apes, is due to genes that affect the cells of the neural crest. The cells of this necklace-shaped structure in the young embryo migrate to become elements of the autonomic nervous system, sensory ganglia, and the melanocytes responsible for the pigmentation of the skin and iris. Variation in these structures has implications for human functioning. For example, European-Caucasians with light blue eyes are more vulnerable to alcohol abuse than those with dark eyes (Sulovari, Kranzler,Farrer, Gelernter, & Li, 2015). Children born with a parasympathetic system that generates high vagal tone are protected from anxiety (Kagan & Snidman, 2004).

Charles Darwin, who was careful in the language he used in his famous 1859 book on the origin of species, was less cautious a dozen years later when he wrote *The Descent of Man, and Selection in Relation to Sex* (Darwin,1871). Darwin attributed reason, happiness, courage, love, ennui, and grief to a variety of animal species and described one baboon as possessing a "capacious heart." This habit remains strong.

The recent suggestion that bonobo chimps are sensitive to the emotions of others was based on faster response times to touch the side of the screen where a picture of a bonobo yawning, grooming another, or engaging in sex appeared than at the side where a different picture was illustrated (called the dot probe paradigm). However, the same bonobos did not display fast response times to pictures of bonobos in a distress state and showed equally fast response times to non-emotional pictures of sheep and rabbits (Kret, Jaasma, Bionda, & Wijnen, 2016). More important, the picture that produced the fastest response times showed a bonobo revealing its large canine teeth in a yawn. Because the teeth were the source of a large contrast in luminance, the fast latencies were most likely due to this feature and did not reflect empathy.

The practice of borrowing concepts with distinctive meanings and validities when they refer to human psychological processes and applying them to brains or animals is reminiscent of the labels early-nineteenth-century phrenologists gave to locations on the skull. Memory, language, and a sense of time were assigned to the frontal lobe; self-esteem to the parietal cortex; and acquisitiveness to the temporal lobe (Combe, 1851). Goethe recognized the danger of assuming that a popular word probably named a natural event. He phrased this danger over 225 years ago, "A physicist … must avoid turning the perception into concepts, the concepts into words, and treating these words as if they were objects" (Bell, 2016, pp. 952–953).

Study Puzzling Events—Avoid Proving the Reality of Words

Searching for the conditions responsible for puzzling phenomena is an alternative to finding the brain sites that represent popular concepts (Izquierdo, Furini, & Myskiw, 2016; Yanai & Lercher, 2016). The molecular biologists who made the surprising discovery that noncoding RNA sequences regulate gene expression did not begin their inquiries by looking for the causes of gene regulation. Rather, they probed the structure and functions of varied RNA forms.

The most frequently cited papers on neuroimaging report a new technology that measures the brain more accurately, rather than describe an attempt to confirm an a priori hypothesis (Kim, Yoon, Kim, Lee, Bae, & Lee, 2016). A research strategy that begins with curiosity about a reliable but puzzling phenomenon will prove to be more profitable than one that selects a word, such as neuroticism, regulation, or reward, and searches for its instantiation in the brain.

The endocrinologists and behavioral biologists of the 1950s would have taken far longer to discover the cascade that leads to masculinization of the brain of the vertebrate male embryo if they had begun with a favorite concept. They were surprised to learn that the enzyme aromatase converted testicular androgens into estradiol which, by activating estrogen receptors in the brain, masculinized sites in the developing brain of a male rat or mouse (McCarthy, 2011). It is unlikely that any nineteenth-century scientist would have imagined this cascade. The concepts of proton, neutron, and electron were invented, after the fact, to explain patterns of evidence. Ernest Rutherford did not first posit an atomic nucleus and try to confirm the reality of this entity with experimental data. Rather, he inferred it from unexpected observations. The zoo of particles that existed before Gell-Mann introduced the concept of quarks were inferences from data on the interactions of various kinds of energy.

The success of this strategy in physics implies that neuroscientists should examine the brain profiles, across all sites, that accompany varied types of incentives and invent constructs that account for the robust regularities. For example, it should be profitable to record the pattern of voxels activated in adults asked to recall a series of 10 unrelated words, 10 unrelated scenes, and 10 unrelated numbers after a 5 second delay and determine whether one, two or three concepts are needed to explain the data. This approach may prove to be more promising than positing the construct of short memory and examining activity in a restricted set of sites in the service of confirming the construct. The neuroscientists who prefer to confirm a favored theoretical idea have forgotten that the powerful theories of modern physics were preceded by many unexpected discoveries. Even Einstein needed the evidence on redshift values and the precession of planetary orbits in order to arrive at the equations of General Relativity.

Hundreds of studies involving several thousand scientists who spent millions of dollars have proceeded from the premise that the abstract concept of neuroticism was a natural kind. The investigators who have been looking for the alleles that accompanied a score on a questionnaire ignored the fact that identical scores can be the result of different biological and experiential conditions. Not surprisingly, these scientists did not find any allele that made a substantial contribution to neuroticism. They might have been more successful if they had selected phenomena that were more likely to be natural kinds. They could have looked for adults who combined a report of frequent feelings of uncertainty with a large rise in heart rate, a decrease in heart rate variability, and increased tension in the corrugator muscle when anticipating criticism for a poor performance, and searched for the alleles associated with this pattern of measures.

A search for the brain circuit that mediates fear in a rat—a mission that can be traced to a 1951 study of potentiated startle in that species (Brown, Kalish, & Farber, 1951)—differs from a search for the brain circuit that mediates freezing, startle, or flight to a conditioned signal for shock. The research in my laboratory that led to the fruitful concepts of high- and low-reactive infants originated in the robust observation that about 20 percent of two-year-old children were unusually cautious and restrained in unfamiliar settings or with unfamiliar people and a larger group was very bold. We set out to discover the origins of these two patterns of behaviors. Had my colleagues and I decided that variation in intensity of fear was the basis for the different behaviors, we would not have discovered these two temperamental biases.

The Main Theme

The point of this chapter is that many predicates that are appropriate when a human is the agent are inappropriate descriptors for a brain profile or the actions of an animal. This issue was the focus of a debate between Maxwell Bennett, a neuroscientist, and Peter Hacker, a philosopher, who objected to the practice of using predicates implying psychological processes in sentences in which the brain was the noun. Daniel Dennett and John Searle saw nothing wrong with this habit (Bennett, Dennett, Hacker, & Searle, 2007). Dennett and Searle argued that it was legitimate to write that "the hippocampus remembers a name" because neuroscientists understood this statement to mean that activity in the hippocampus contributes to and is necessary for remembering a name. Because neuroscientists agree on the meaning of "remember" in the above sentence, it is not an error to attribute psychological properties to the brain. This position is reasonable when the language community consists only of neuroscientists. But there is the potential for misunderstanding when others read the same sentence. That is why Le Doux (2014) and Le Doux and Pine (2016) suggested that the term *fear* presupposes a conscious human agent and should not be used to describe a brain profile, a startle, freezing, or the avoidance of a lit alley or center of an open arena. Sixty years earlier Solomon and Wynne (1953) selected the term *emotional*, rather than fear, to describe the state of a dog that was reluctant to enter a section of a chamber where it had been shocked.

Consider an observation that has been interpreted as reflecting fear. A rat is placed in a white chamber that is separated from a black chamber by a gate. Because rats prefer dark to light, the rat moves to the black chamber when the gate is raised. Once in the black chamber the animal receives an electric shock. When the rat is placed in the white chamber the next day it does not immediately move to the black one. This delay was interpreted as reflecting a state of fear.

It is reasonable to argue that the setting triggered an anticipation of the unpleasant feeling of electric shock in the black chamber. The resulting brain state activated the central nucleus of the amygdala, which sent GABAergic projections to the ventrolateral column of the central gray, which in turn removed the GABAergic inhibition on the neurons that cause freezing. Once these neurons are freed from their inhibited state, the animal becomes immobile. These three sentences explain the evidence without using the word *fear*. The reasonableness of this argument is revealed in the observation that female rhesus macaque monkeys with low levels of cortisol in their hair, compared with animals with high concentrations of hair cortisol, spent more time freezing but less time in the back of their cage when a human intruder stared at them (Hamel, Lutz, Coleman, Worlein, Peterson, Rosenberg et al., 2017). This result implies that freezing does not always reflect a state of fear. Adolphs, Kretch, & LoBue (2014) make the same point in discussing infants' reluctance to crawl over a piece of glass that evokes the perception of a drop-off, called a visual cliff. The avoidant behavior does not necessarily reflect a state of fear. About six months ago I tripped on the bottom stair of the stairwell in my home as I descended from the second to the first floor. Ever since that time I automatically slow down as I approach the bottom stair. My state is best described as attentive or vigilant, rather than fear.

Nonetheless, scientists who work with mice or rats as models for human anxiety disorders continue to interpret an animal's avoidance of the center of an arena as a sign of anxiety (Li, Nakajima, Ibanez-Tallon, & Heintz, 2016). The adults who avoid spicy foods or large cities do so because they do not like the sensations these experiences generate. They do not interpret these feelings as implying a threat to their welfare and, therefore, would not say they are anxious when they refuse a spicy food at a dinner party or refuse an opportunity to visit Los Angeles. The rats who avoid the center of an arena do so because the sensations are unpleasant, not because they are fearful or anxious (Ennaceur & Chazot, 2016).

The practice of awarding terms naming psychological phenomena to brain profiles or animals is reminiscent of Humpty Dumpty's declaration that a word means whatever he says it means (Parkinson & Haggard, 2015; Jensen, Kaptchuk, Chen, Kirsch, Ingvar, Gollub, & Kong, 2015; Palombo, Keane, & Verfaellie, 2016; Strawson, 2013). The mathematician Frank Ramsey captured the dangers lurking in this practice in a pithy sentence: "What we can't say, we can't say, and we can't whistle it either" (Mellor, 1990).

7 Coda

This review of some of the reasons why the pace of progress in the study of brain–behavior relations has been slower than many anticipated is not meant to imply that brain evidence is of minimal value in attempts to understand mental processes. Rather, the aim is quite the opposite. I wanted to document the value of gathering patterns of measures representing possible causes of outcomes and evaluating their predictive power with patterns of measures, many of which should be brain profiles.

Investigators should gather as many different sources of evidence as they can because a variable thought to be irrelevant can be a clue to understanding. Most investigators had interpreted the smaller P3 waveform to deviant visual targets in older adults as a sign of a compromise in brain function. But these scientists had not bothered to assess the adult's visual acuity. A team that did measure visual acuity found that it was the older adults with poor acuity who showed the smaller P3 waveform (Porto, Tusch, Fox, Alperin, Holcomb, & Daffner, 2016).

If measures of each subject's social class, vocabulary, ethnicity, height, weight, facial width, hair and eye color, and sitting and standing heart rate, heart rate variability, and blood pressure were gathered regularly and added to the variables of interest, investigators might uncover important and surprising facts. Because Nancy Snidman and I did include some of these variables in our research on temperament we learned that Caucasian children with narrow faces, blue eyes, an ectomorphic body build, and a high and minimally variable heart rate were prone to withdraw from unexpected or unfamiliar events (Kagan & Snidman, 2004).

I also wanted to provoke brooding over an imbalance in the study of brain–behavior relations that favors experiments designed to affirm a favored, a priori hypothesis over attempts to illuminate a puzzling observation. Consider three robust, important phenomena in search of a deeper understanding. What patterns of experiences and biology render a child's social class such a powerful predictor of so many adult outcomes? What are the distinctive patterns of genes, experiences, and brain measures that that characterize the symptoms defining each of the DSM categories of mental illness? What maturational changes in the brain allow the emergence of speech, inference, and a moral sense in the second year? Balancing the current preference for hypothesis-driven experiments with a Baconian strategy that seeks to shed light on an obvious and important puzzle is likely to yield significant advances in the understanding of brain–behavior relations.

Many influential discoveries in psychology were unexpected. Five examples are Ivan Pavlov's discovery of conditioned salivation, Harry Harlow's noting the odd behaviors of infant monkeys raised apart from the mother, James Olds's recordings of pleasure sites in the brain, James Robertson's observation of the distress of a two-year-old on a hospital ward, which was the source of John Bowlby's ideas on attachment, and Roger Brown's discovery of the sequence of acquisition of grammatical forms in three children learning English.

Many of the scientists celebrated in textbooks—Kepler, Harvey, Mendel, Darwin, Pasteur, the Curies, Fermi, Crick and Watson, Barr, and McClintock—tried to understand a robust phenomenon rather than prove a favorite idea. David Hubel and Torsten Wiesel (2005) confessed that they had no hypothesis when they began to record neural activity in the visual cortex of a cat. It was, they admitted, a fishing expedition. Georg von Bekesy, awarded a Nobel Prize in 1961 for research on the basilar membrane, took Leonardo da Vinci as a model because this artist tried to learn from nature rather than dictate its properties.

Geneticists were surprised to learn that only 2 percent of the human genome code for proteins while 80 percent regulate the expression of these genes. No biologist would have predicted that fact 60 years ago. Lily and Yuh Nung Jan, who discovered the first potassium channel gene, bemoaned the pressure on young biologists to implement hypothesis driven studies that restrict the operation of serendipity. The confirmation of a significant idea usually follows the gathering of a corpus of data large and reliable enough to generate a significant theoretical proposition. Several decades of careful research on the atom had to precede Enrico Fermi's insight that neutrons aimed at a target had to be slowed, by placing the apparatus on paraffin, in order to induce radioactivity in the target. Many domains in psychology and neuroscience have not reached a phase of maturity that permits major insights. Psychologists and neuroscientists need a richer collection of facts before testing the theoretical power of most a priori ideas concerned with emotions, thoughts, and beliefs.

The research posture advocated here requires neuroscientists and psychologists to be more concerned than they have been with the features in the laboratory setting, the details in the procedure, the participants' expectations, the specific evidence cited as the basis for an inference, and the vocabulary used to describe a brain or behavioral outcome. The current search for reliable relations among genes, experiences, brain profiles, mental processes, and behaviors remains in an early stage. A patient probing of puzzling phenomena has proven to be a more profitable strategy in young disciplines than attempts to confirm abstract theoretical ideas that are silent on the circumstances.

Paul Volcker is fond of a joke that satirizes the economists' attraction to abstract mathematical theory that ignores the constraints contexts impose. A squirrel who wished to add fish to his diet consulted a wise owl in order to learn how to satisfy his desire. The owl thought a long time before telling the squirrel that he should scamper up a tree by a lake and imagine being a kingfisher. The squirrel took the advice but after several months of failure returned to the owl to complain. The owl, irritated by the squirrel's criticism, replied angrily, "You came to me with a problem. I gave you what I believed was a useful policy recommendation. The rest is operational detail." A paraphrase of a comment by Bertrand Russell in 1918 captures the current state of affairs in study of brain–mind relations and provides a good way to end this narrative. The statement that the brain is the foundation of all psychological events is so obviously true it does not need repeating. The paradox lies in our inability to explain how the properties of this materialistic structure could be the origin of phenomena that, at the moment, seem to bear little relation to their source.

References

Adolphs, K. E., Kretch, K. S., & LoBue, V. (2014). Fear of heights in infants? *Current Directions in Psychological Science, 23*, 60–66.

Albertazzi, L., Da Pos, O., Canal, L., Micciolo, R., Malfatti, M., & Vescovi, M. (2013). The hue of shapes. *Journal of Experimental Psychology: Human Perception and Performance, 39*, 37–47.

Albright, T. D. (2015). Perceiving. *Daedalus, 144*, 22–41.

Aldridge, K. (2011). Patterns of differences in brain morphology in humans as compared to extant apes. *Journal of Human Evolution, 60*, 94–105.

Alexander, G. M., & Hines, M. (2002). Sex differences in response to children's toys in nonhuman primates (*Cercopithecus aethiops sabaeus*). *Evolution and Human Behavior, 23*, 467–479.

Al-Hashim, A. H., Blaser, S., Raybaud, C., & MacGregor, D. (2016). Corpus callosum abnormalities. *Developmental Medicine and Child Neurology, 58*, 475–484.

Alkozei, A., Smith, R. S., & Killgore, W. D. (2016). Exposure to blue wavelength light modulates Anterior cingulate cortex activation in response to 'uncertain' versus 'certain' anticipation of positive stimuli. *Neuroscience Letters, 11*, 5–10.

Almeida, I., Soares, S. C., & Castelo-Branco, M. (2015). The distinct role of the amygdala, superior colliculus and pulvinar in processing of central and peripheral snakes. *PLoS One, 10*, e0129949.

Amado, C., Hermann, P., Kovacs, M., Grotheer, M., Vidnyanszky, Z., & Kovacs, G. (2016). The contribution of surprise to the prediction-based modulation of fMRI responses. *Neuropsychologia, 84,* 105–112.

Amaral, D. G., & Adolphs, R. (Eds.). (2016). *Living without an amygdala.* New York: The Guilford Press.

Ames, D. L., & Fiske, S. T. (2013). Intentional harms are worse, even when they're not. *Psychological Science, 24,* 1755–1762.

Aminoff, E. M., Kveraga, K., & Bar, M. (2013). The role of the parahippocampal cortex in cognition. *Trends in Cognitive Sciences, 17,* 379–390.

Amsel, B. D., DeLong, K. A., & Kutas, M. (2015). Close, but no garlic: Perceptuomotor and event knowledge activation during language comprehension. *Journal of Memory and Language, 82,* 118–132.

Amunts, K., Armstrong, E., Malikovic, A., Homke, L., Mohlberg, H., Schleicher, A., & Zilles, K. (2007). Gender-specific left-right asymmetries in human visual cortex. *Journal of Neuroscience, 27,* 1356–1364.

Andreatta, M., Leombruni, E., Glotzbach-Schoon, E., Pauli, P., & Muhlberger, A. (2015). Generalization of contextual fear in humans. *Behavior Therapy, 46,* 583–596.

Andrillon, T., Poulsen, A. T., Hansen, L. K., Leger, D., & Kouider, S. (2016). Neural markers of responsiveness to the environment in human sleep. *Journal of Neuroscience, 36,* 6583–6596.

Arditte, K. A., Cek, D., Shaw, A. M., & Timpano, K. R. (2016). The importance of assessing clinical phenomena in Mechanical Turk research. *Psychological Assessment, 28,* 684–691.

Arpawong, T. E., Lee, J., Phillips, D. F., Crimmins, E. M., Levine, M. E., & Prescott, C. A. (2016). Effects of recent stress and variation in the serotonin transporter polymorphism (5-HTTLPR) on depressive symptoms. *Behavior Genetics, 46,* 72–88.

Axelrod, V. (2016). On the domain-specificity of the visual and non-visual face-selective regions. *European Journal of Neuroscience, 44,* 2049–2063.

Babo-Rebelo, M., Richter, C. G., & Tallon-Baudry, C. (2016). Neural responses to heartbeats in the default network encode the self in spontaneous thoughts. *Journal of Neuroscience*, *36*, 7829–7840.

Bachevalier, J., Sanchez, M., Raper, J., Stephens, S. B. Z., & Wallen, K. (2016). The effects of neonatal amygdala lesions in Rhesus monkeys living in a species-typical social environment. In D. G. Amaral & R. Adolphs (Eds.), *Living without an amygdala*, 186–217. New York: The Guilford Press.

Bakken, T. E., Miller, J. A., Ding, S. L., Sunkin, S. M., Smith, K. A., Ng, L., et al. (2016). A comprehensive transcriptional map of primate brain development. *Nature*, *535*, 367–375.

Balaban, H., & Luria, R. (2016). Object representations in visual working memory change according to the task context. *Cortex*, *81*, 1–13.

Balconi, M., & Cortesi, L. (2015). Brain activity (fNIRS) in control state differs from the execution and observation of object-related and object-unrelated actions. *Journal of Motor Behavior*, *16*, 1–18.

Balderston, N. L., Schultz, D. H., & Helmstetter, F. J. (2011). The human amygdala plays a stimulus specific role in the detection of novelty. *NeuroImage*, *55*, 1889–1898.

Balderston, N. L., Schultz, D. H., Hopkins, L., & Helmstetter, F. J. (2015). Functionally distinct amygdala subregions identified using DTI and high resolution fMRI. *Social Cognitive and Affective Neuroscience*, *10*, 1615–1622.

Bambini, V., Resta, D., & Grimaldi, M. (2014). A dataset of metaphors from the Italian literature. *PLoS One*, *9*, e105634.

Bar, M., Aminoff, E., & Ishai, A. (2008). Famous faces activate contextual associations in the parahippocampal cortex. *Cerebral Cortex*, *18*, 1233–1238.

Bar, M., & Neta, M. (2007). Visual elements of subjective preference modulate amygdala activation. *Neuropsychologia*, *45*, 2191–2200.

Barascud, N., Pearce, M. T., Griffiths, T. D., Friston, K. J., & Chait, M. (2016). Brain responses in humans reveal ideal observer-like sensitivity to complex acoustic patterns. *Proceedings of the National Academy of Sciences of the United States of America, 113*, E616–E625.

Barger, B., Nabi, R., & Hong, L. Y. (2010). Standard back-translation procedures may not capture proper emotion concepts. *Emotion, 10*, 703–711.

Barger, N., Stefanacci, L., & Semendeferi, K. (2007). A comparative volumetric analysis of the amygdaloid complex and basolateral division in the human and ape brain. *American Journal of Physical Anthropology, 134*, 392–403.

Barrett, H. C., Bolyanatz, A., Crittenden, A. N., Fessler, D. M. T., Fitzpatrick, S., Gurven, M., et al. (2016). Small-scale societies exhibit variation in the role of intentions in moral judgment. *Proceedings of the National Academy of Sciences of the United States of America, 113*, 4688–4693.

Barth, C., Villringer, A., & Sacher, J. (2015). Sex hormones affect neurotransmitters and shape the adult female brain during hormonal transition periods. *Frontiers in Neuroscience, 9*, 37–44.

Bartoshuk, L. (2014). The measurement of pleasure and pain. *Perspectives on Psychological Science, 9*, 91–93.

Bartz, J. A. (2016). Oxytocin and the pharmacological dissection of affiliation. *Current Directions in Psychological Science, 25*, 104–110.

Baumann, O., Borra, R. J., Bower, J. M., Cullen, K. E., Habas, C., Ivry, R. B., et al. (2015). Consensus paper: The role of the cerebellum in perceptual processes. *The Cerebellum, 14*, 197–220.

Bayne, T., Hohwy, J., & Owen, A. M. (2016). Are there levels of consciousness? *Trends in Cognitive Sciences, 20*, 405–413.

Beisner, B. A., Jin, J., Fushing, H., & Mccowan, B. (2015). Detection of social group instability among captive rhesus macaques using joint network modeling. *Current Zoology, 61*, 70–84.

Bekar, L. K., Wei, H. S., & Nedergaard, M. (2012). The locus coeruleus-norepinephrine network optimizes coupling of cerebral blood volume with oxygen demand. *Journal of Cerebral Blood Flow and Metabolism, 32*, 2135–2145.

Bekhuis, E., Boschloo, L., Rosmalen, J. G. M., de Boer, M. K., & Schoevers, R. A. (2016). The impact of somatic symptoms on the course of major depressive disorder. *Journal of Affective Disorders, 205*, 112–118.

Bell, M. (Ed.). (2016). *The essential Goethe.* Princeton, NJ: Princeton University Press.

Belova, M. A., Paton, J. J., Morrison, S. E., & Salzman, C. D. (2007). Expectation modulates neural responses to pleasant and aversive stimuli in primate amygdala. *Neuron, 55*, 970–984.

Benenson, J. F., Tennyson, R., & Wrangham, R. W. (2011). More male than female infants imitate propulsive motion. *Cognition, 121*, 262–267.

Bennett, M., Dennett, D., Hacker, P., & Searle, J. (2007). *Neuroscience and philosophy.* New York: Columbia University Press.

Bentin, S., Golland, Y., Flevaris, A., Robertson, L. C., & Moscovitch, M. (2006). Processing the trees and the forest during initial stages of face perception. *Journal of Cognitive Neuroscience, 18*, 1406–1425.

Beran, M. J., James, B. T., Whithan, W., & Parrish, A. E. (2016). Chimpanzees can point to smaller amounts of food to accumulate larger amounts but they still fail the reverse-reward contingency task. *Journal of Experimental Psychology. Animal Learning and Cognition, 42*, 347–358.

Beran, M. J., & Parrish, A. E. (2016). Going for more. In A. Henik (Ed.), *Continuous issues in numerical cognition* (pp. 177–195). New York: Elsevier.

Berenbaum, S. A., & Beltz, A. M. (2016). How early hormones shape gender development. *Current Opinion in Behavioral Sciences, 7*, 53–60.

Bergman, L. R. (1998). A pattern-oriented approach to studying individual development. In R. B. Cairns, L. R. Bergman, & J. Kagan (Eds.),

Methods and models for studying the individual (pp. 83–101). Thousand Oaks, CA: Sage.

Betancourt, L. M., Avants, B., Farah, M. J., Brodsky, N. L., Wu, J., Ashtari, M., et al. (2016). Effect of socioeconomic status (SES) disparity on neural development in female African-American infants at age 1 month. *Developmental Science*, *19*, 947–956.

Biagioli, M. (2016). Watch out for cheats in citation game. *Nature*, *535*, 201.

Bilalic, M. (2016). Revisiting the role of the fusiform face area in expertise. *Journal of Cognitive Neuroscience*, *28*, 1345–1357.

Bilalic, M., Grottenthaler, T., Nagele, T., & Lindig, T. (2016). The faces in radiological images. *Cerebral Cortex*, *26*, 1004–1014.

Bizzi, E., Cheung, V. C. K., d'Avella, P., Saltiel, P., & Tresch, M. (2008). Combining modules for movement. *Brain Research. Brain Research Reviews*, *57*, 125–133.

Bleidorn, W., Arslan, R. C., Denisson, J. J. A., Rentfrow, P. T., Gebaver, J. E., Potter, J., & Gosling, S. D. (2016). Age and gender differences in self-esteem. *Journal of Personality and Social Psychology*, *111*, 396–410.

Bockhorst, T., & Himberg, U. (2015). Compass cells in the brain of an insect are sensitive to novel events in the visual world. *PLoS One*, *10*, e0144501.

Bodde, D. (1991). *Chinese thought, society, and science*. Honolulu: University of Hawaii Press.

Boden, J. M., van Stockum, S., Horwood, L. J., & Fergusson, D. M. (2016). Bullying victimization in adolescence and psychotic symptomatology in adulthood. *Psychological Medicine*, *46*, 1311–1320.

Boehm, L. K., & Corey, S. H. (2015). *America's urban history*. New York: Routledge.

Bonner, M. F., Peelle, J. E., Cook, P. A., & Grossman, M. (2013). Heteromodal conceptual processing in the angular gyrus. *NeuroImage*, *71*, 175–186.

Booth-LaForce, C., & Roisman, G. I. (2014). The adult attachment interview: Psychometrics, stability and change from infancy, and developmental origins. *Monographs of the Society for Research in Child Development, 79*(3), 1–185.

Borg, C., Georgiadis, J. R., Renken, R. J., Spoelstra, S. K., Weijmar-Schultz, W., & de Jong, P. J. (2014). Brain processing of visual stimuli representing sexual penetration versus core and animal-reminder disgust in women with lifelong vaginismus. *PLoS One, 9*, e84882. doi:10.1371.

Bornstein, M. H., Putnick, D. L., Lansford, J. E., Deater-Deckard, K., & Bradley, R. H. (2016). Gender in low- and middle-income countries. *Monographs of the Society for Research in Child Development, 81*, 1–170.

Bowlby, J. (1950). *Attachment and loss* (Vol. 1). New York: Basic Books.

Bracci, S., Caramazza, A., & Peelen, M. V. (2015). Representational similarity of body parts in human occipitotemporal cortex. *Journal of Neuroscience, 35*, 12977–12985.

Bracci, S., & Op de Beeck, H. (2016). Dissociations and associations between shape and category representations in the two visual pathways. *Journal of Neuroscience, 36*, 432–444.

Bradford, D. E., Kaye, J. T., & Curtin, J. J. (2014). Not just noise: Individual differences in general startle reactivity predict startle response to uncertain and certain threat. *Psychophysiology, 51*, 407–411.

Bradley, M. M., Lang, P. J., & Cuthbert, B. N. (1993). Emotion, novelty, and the startle reflex. *Behavioral Neuroscience, 107*, 970–980.

Brandon, M. P., Koenig, J., & Leutgeb, S. (2014). Parallel and convergent processing in grid cell, head-direction cell, boundary cell, and place cell networks. *Wiley Interdisciplinary Reviews: Cognitive Science, 5*, 207–219.

Brandt, D. J., Sommer, J., Krach, S., Bedenbender, J., Kircher, T., Paulus, F. M., & Jansen, A. (2013). Test-retest reliability of fMRI brain activity during memory encoding. *Frontiers in Psychiatry, 4*, 163. doi:10.3389/fpsyt.2013.00163.

Bravo-Rivera, C., Diehl, M. M., Roman-Ortiz, C., Rodriguez-Romaguera, J., Rosas-Vidal, L. E., Bravo-Rivera, H., et al. (2015). Long-range GABAergic neurons in the prefrontal cortex modulate behavior. *Journal of Neurophysiology*, *114*, 1357–1363.

Bredewold, R., Smith, C. J., Dumais, K. M., & Veenema, A. H. (2014). Sex-specific modulation of juvenile social play behavior by vasopressin and oxytocin depends on social context. *Frontiers in Behavioral Neuroscience*, *8*, 216.

Brendgen, M., Girard, A., Vitaro, F., Dionne, G., & Boivin, M. (2016). Personal and familial predictors of peer victimization trajectories from primary to secondary school. *Developmental Psychology*, *52*, 1103–1114.

Brown, J. S., Kalish, H. I., & Farber, I. E. (1951). Conditioned fear as revealed by magnitude of startle response to an auditory stimulus. *Journal of Experimental Psychology*, *41*, 317–328.

Brown, R. (1958). *Words and things*. Glencoe, IL: The Free Press.

Bruckner, P. (2010). *The tyranny of guilt* (S. Rendall, Trans.). Princeton, NJ: Princeton University Press.

Buchanan, T. (2016). Self-report measures of executive function problems correlate with personality, not performance-based executive function measures, in nonclinical samples. *Psychological Assessment*, *28*, 372–385.

Buckingham, G., Goodale, M. A., White, J. A., & Westwood, D. A. (2016). Equal-magnitude size-weight illusions experienced within and between object categories. *Journal of Vision*, *16*(3), 25. doi:10.1167/16.3.25.

Bueti, D., & Macaluso, E. (2010). Auditory temporal expectations modulate activity in visual cortex. *NeuroImage*, *51*, 1168–1183.

Bulthe, J., De Smedt, B., & Op de Beeck, H. P. (2015). Visual number beats abstract numerical magnitude. *Journal of Cognitive Neuroscience*, *27*, 1376–1387.

Bunzeck, N., Guitart-Massip, M., Dolan, R. J., & Duzel, E. (2014). Pharmacological dissociation of novelty responses in the human brain. *Cerebral Cortex*, *24*, 1351–1360.

Burakevych, N., McKinlay, C. J., Alsweiler, J. M., Harding, J. E., & CHYLD Study Team. (2015). Accuracy of caregivers' recall of hospital admissions: Implications for research. *Acta Paediatrica*, *104*, 1199–1204.

Burra, N., Hervais-Adelman, A., Kerzel, D., Tamietto, M., de Gelder, B., & Pegna, A. J. (2013). Amygdala activation for eye contact despite complete cortical blindness. *Journal of Neuroscience*, *33*, 10483–10489.

Buxton, R. B. (2013). The physics of functional magnetic resonance imaging (fMRI). *Reports on Progress in Physics*, *76*(9).

Buzsaki, G. (2016). Q & A. *Neuron*, *91*, 217.

Byrd, A. L., Hawes, S. W., Loeber, R., & Pardini, D. A. (2016). Interpersonal callousness from childhood to adolescence. *Journal of Clinical Child and Adolescent Psychology*, *21*, 1–16.

Caldera, R., Seghier, M. L., Rossion, B., Lazeyras, F., Michel, C., & Hauert, C. A. (2006). The fusiform face area is tuned for curvilinear patterns with more high-contrasted elements in the upper part. *NeuroImage*, *31*, 313–319.

Calderon, D. P., Kilinc. M., Maritan, A., Banaver, J., & Pfaff, D. (2016). Generalized CNS arousal: An elementary force within the vertebrate nervous system. *Neuroscience and Biobehavioral Reviews*, May 20. pii:S0149–7634(15)30356–0.

Calvo, M. G., Avero, P., Fernandez-Martin, A., & Recio, G. (2016). Recognition thresholds for static and dynamic emotional faces. *Emotion*, *16*, 1186–1200.

Caminiti, R., Chafee, M. V., Battaglia-Mayer, A., Averbach, B. B., Crowe, D. A., & Georgopoulos, A. P. (2010). Understanding the parietal lobe syndrome from a neurophysiological and evolutionary perspective. *European Journal of Neuroscience*, *31*, 2310–2340.

Campo, R. A., Light, K. C., O'Connor, K., Nakamura, Y., Lipschitz, D., La Stayo, P. C., et al. (2015). Blood pressure, salivary cortisol, and inflammatory cytokine outcomes in senior female cancer survivors enrolled in a tai chi chih randomized controlled trial. *Journal of Cancer Survivorship: Research and Practice, 9*, 115–125.

Canario, N., Jorge, L., Silva, M. F. L., Soares, M. A., & Castelo-Branco, M. (2016). Distinct preference for spatial frequency content in ventral stream regions underlying the recognition of scenes, faces, bodies, and other objects. *Neuropsychologia, 87*, 110–119.

Canetta, S., Bolkan, S., Padilla-Coreano, N., Song, L. J., Sahn, R., Harrison, N. L., et al. (2016). Maternal immune activation leads to selective functional deficits in offspring parvalbumin interneurons. *Molecular Psychiatry, 21*, 956–968.

Cantrell, L., & Smith, L. B. (2013). Open questions and a proposal. *Cognition, 128*, 331–352.

Cao, J., & Banaji, M. R. (2016). The base rate principle and the fairness principle in social judgment. *Proceedings of the National Academy of Sciences of the United States of America, 113*, 7475–7480.

Carey, S. (2009). *The origin of concepts.* New York: Oxford University Press.

Casey, B. J., & Caudle, K. (2013). The teenage brain: Self control. *Current Directions in Psychological Science, 22*, 82–87.

Catena, A., Perales, J. C., Megias, A., Candido, A., Jara, E., & Maldonado, A. (2012). The brain network of expectancy and uncertainty processing. *PLoS One, 7*, e40252.

Centers for Disease Control and Prevention. (2007). *State-based prevalence data of ADHD diagnosis.* Atlanta, GA.

Chan, C. H., Caine, E. D., You, S., & Yip, P. S. (2015). Changes in South Korean urbanicity and suicide rates, 1992 to 2012. *BMJ Open, 5*(12) e009451. doi:10.1136/bmjopen-2015-009451.

Chang, C., Metzger, C. D., Glover, G. H., Duyn, J. H., Heinze, H. J., & Walter, M. (2012). Association between heart rate variability and fluctuations in resting-state functional connectivity. *NeuroImage*, *68*, 93–100.

Chen, S. X., Benet-Martinez, V., & Ng, J. C. (2014). Does language affect personality perception? *Journal of Personality*, *82*, 130–143.

Chen, X., Hackett, P. D., DeMarco, A. C., Feng, C., Stair, S., Haroon, E., et al. (2015). Effects of oxytocin and vasopressin on the neural responses to unreciprocated cooperation within brain regions involved in stress and anxiety in men and women. *Brain Imaging and Behavior*, *9*, 754–764.

Chen, J. Y. C., & Mazzocco, M. M. M. (2017). Competing features influence children's attention to number. *Journal of Experimental Child Psychology*, *156*, 62–81.

Chestnut, E. K., & Markman, E. M. (2016). Are horses like zebras, or vice versa? Children's sensitivity to the asymmetries of directional comparisons. *Child Development*, *87*, 568–582.

Chmielewski, M., Clark, L. A., Bagby, R. M., & Watson, D. (2015). Method matters. *Journal of Abnormal Psychology*, *124*, 764–769.

Chou, M. Y., Amo, R., Kinoshita, M., Cherng, B. W., Shimazaki, H., Agetsuma, M., et al. (2016). Social conflict resolution regulated by two dorsal habenular subregions in zebrafish. *Science*, *352*, 87–90.

Christie, S., Gentner, D., Call, J., Benjamin, D., & Haun, D. B. M. (2016). Sensitivity to relational similarity and object similarity in apes and children. *Current Biology*, *26*, 531–535.

Chua, H. F., Boland, J. E., & Nisbett, R. E. (2005). Cultural variation in eye movements during scene perception. *Proceedings of the National Academy of Sciences of the United States of America*, *102*, 12629–12633.

Church, A. T., Alvarez, J. M., Mai, N. T. Q., French, B. F., Katigbak, M. S., & Ortiz, F. A. (2011). Are cross-cultural comparisons of personality profiles meaningful? *Journal of Personality and Social Psychology*, *101*, 1068–1089.

Churchland, P. S., & Winkielman, P. (2012). Modulating social behavior with oxytocin. *Hormones and Behavior, 61*, 392–399.

Civile, C., & Obhi, S. (2016). Power eliminates the influence of body posture on facial emotion recognition. *Journal of Nonverbal Behavior, 40*, 283–289.

Clark, B. C., Mahato, N. K., Nakazawa, M., Law, T. D., & Thomas, J. S. (2014). The power of the mind. *Journal of Neurophysiology, 113*, 3219–3226.

Clark, B. J., & Harvey, R. E. (2016). Do the anterior and lateral thalamic nuclei make distinct contributions to spatial representations and memory? *Neurobiology of Learning and Memory, 133*, 69–78.

Clark, D. A., Listro, C. J., Lo, S. L., Durbin, C. E., Donnellan, M. B., & Neppl, T. K. (2016). Measurement invariance and child temperament. *Psychological Assessment, 28*, 1646–1662.

Clark, S. (2016). *The unknown universe*. New York: Pegasus Books.

Clark-Polner, E., Johnson, T. D., & Barrett, L. F. (2016). Multivoxel pattern analysis does not provide evidence to support the existence of basic emotions. *Cerebral Cortex* , doi:10.1093/cercor/bhw028.

Clay, Z., Ravaux, L., de Waal, F. B. M., & Zuberbuhler, K. (2016). Bonobos (*Pan paniscus*) vocally protest against violations of social expectations. *Journal of Comparative Psychology, 130*, 44–54.

Clifford, S., Lemery-Chalfant, K., & Goldsmith, H. H. (2015). The unique and shared genetic and environmental contributions to fear, anger, and sadness in childhood. *Child Development, 86*, 1538–1556.

Cloutier, J., Gabrieli, J. D., O'Young, D., & Ambady, N. (2011). An fMRI study of violation of social expectations. *NeuroImage, 59*, 583–588.

Cogan, D. D., Liu, W., Baker, D. H., & Andrews, T. J. (2016). Category selective patterns of neural response in the ventral visual pathway in the absence of categorical information. *NeuroImage, 135*, 92–106.

Cole, G. G., & Wilkins, A. J. (2013). Fear of holes. *Psychological Science, 94*, 1980–1985.

Coles, M. E., & Ravid, A. (2016). Clinical presentation of not-just right experiences (NJREs) in individuals with OCD. *Behaviour Research and Therapy, 87,* 182–187.

Combe, G. (1851). *A System of Phrenology.* Boston: Benjamin Mussey Publishers.

Compton, W. M., Jones, C. M., & Baldwin, G. T. (2016). Relationship between nonmedical prescription-opioid use and heroin use. *New England Journal of Medicine, 374,* 154–163.

Comte, M., Schon, D., Coull, J. T., Reynaud, E., Khalfa, S., Belzeaux, R., et al. (2016). Dissociating bottom-up and top-down mechanisms in the cortico-limbic system during emotion processing. *Cerebral Cortex, 26,* 144–155.

Connolly, J. D., Kentridge, R. W., & Cavina-Pratesi, C. (2016). Coding of attention across the human intraparietal sulcus. *Experimental Brain Research, 234,* 917–930.

Costa, M., & Bonetti, L. (2016). Geometrical factors in the perception of sacredness. *Perception, 45,* 1240–1256.

Costa, V. D., Dal Monte, O., Lucas, D. R., Murray, E. A., & Averbeck, B. B. (2016). Amygdala and ventral striatum make distinct contributions to reinforcement learning. *Neuron, 92,* 505–517.

Courage, M. L., Reynolds, G. D., & Richards, J. E. (2006). Infants' attention to patterned stimuli. *Child Development, 77,* 680–695.

Cox, D., Meyers, E., & Sinha, P. (2004). Contextually evoked object-specific responses in human visual cortex. *Science, 304,* 115–117.

Crivelli, C., Jarillo, S., Russell, J. A., & Fernandez-Dols, J. M. (2016). Reading emotions from faces in two indigenous societies. *Journal of Experimental Psychology. General, 145,* 830–843.

Crum, K., Cornacchio, D., Coxe, S., Green, J. G., & Comer, J. S. (2016). Conduct problems among Boston-area youth following the 2013 Marathon bombing. *Journal of Clinical Child and Adolescent Psychology, 2,* 1–10.

Dakin, S. C., Tibber, M. S., Greenwood, J. A., Kingdom, F. A. A., & Morgan, M. J. (2011). A common visual metric for approximate number and density. *Proceedings of the National Academy of Sciences of the United States of America, 108,* 19552–19557.

Danto, A. C. (2009). *Andy Warhol.* New. Haven, CT: Yale University Press.

Darwin, C. (1871). *The descent of man and selection in relation to sex* (Vol. 1). London: John Murray.

Daum, M. M., Wronski, C., Harms, A., & Gredebeck, G. (2016). Action perception in infancy. *Experimental Brain Research, 234,* 2465–2478.

Davis, F. C., Neta, M., Kim, M. J., Moran, J. M., & Whalen, P. J. (2016). Interpreting ambiguous social cues in unpredictable contexts. *Social Cognitive and Affective Neuroscience,* Feb 29. pii:nsw003.

Davis, M., & Whalen, P. J. (2001). The amygdala: Vigilance and emotion. *Molecular Psychiatry, 6,* 13–34.

Dean, K., Stevens, H., & Mortensen, P. B. (2010). Full spectrum of psychiatric outcomes among offspring with parental history of mental disorder. *Archives of General Psychiatry, 67,* 822–829.

De Deyne, S., Navarro, D. J., Perfors, A., & Storms, G. (2016). Structure at every scale. *Journal of Experimental Psychology. General, 145,* 1228–1254.

Dehaene, S. (1997). *The Number Sense.* New York: Oxford University Press.

Dehaene, S., Meyniel, F., Wacongne, C., Wang, L., & Pallier, C. (2015). The neural representation of sequences: From transition probabilities to algebraic patterns and linguistic trees. *Neuron, 88,* 2–19.

Denfield, G. H., Fahey, P. G., Reimer, J., & Tolia, A. S. (2016). Investigating the limits of neurovascular coupling. *Neuron, 91,* 954–956.

Depue, B. E., Orr, J. M., Smolker, H. R., Naaz, F., & Banich, M. T. (2016). The organization of right prefrontal networks reveals common mechanisms of inhibitory regulation across cognitive, emotional, and motor processes. *Cerebral Cortex, 26,* 1634–1646.

Desmurget, M., Reilly, K. T., Richard, N., Szathmari, A., Mottolese, C., & Sirigu, A. (2009). Movement intention after parietal cortex stimulation in humans. *Science, 324,* 811–813.

de Vries, Y. A., Roest, A. M., Franzen, M., Munafo, M. R., & Bastiaansen, J. A. (2016). Citation bias and selective focus on positive findings in the literature on the serotonin transporter gene (5-HTTPLR), life stress, and depression. *Psychological Medicine, 46,* 2971–2976.

Dinescu, D., Horn, E. E., Duncan, G., & Turkheimer, E. (2016). Soicoeconomic modifiers of genetic and environmental influences on body mass index in adult twins. *Health Psychology, 35,* 159–161.

Ditz, H. M., & Nieder, A. (2016). Sensory and working memory representations of small and large numerosities in the crow endbrain. *Journal of Neuroscience, 36,* 12044–12052.

Dodge, K. A. (2011). Context matters in child and family policy. *Child Development, 82,* 433–442.

Dorn, L. D., Gayles, J. G., Engelwood, C. G., Houts, R., Cizza, G., & Denson, L. A. (2016). Cytokine patterns in healthy adolescent girls. *Psychosomatic Medicine, 78,* 646–656.

Dreyer, J. K., Vander Weele, C. M., Lovic, V., & Aragona, B. J. (2016). Functionally distinct dopamine signals in nucleus accumbens core and shell in the freely moving rat. *Journal of Neuroscience, 36,* 98–112.

Driver, I. D., Andoh, J., Blockley, N. P., Francis, S. T., Gowland, P. A., & Paus, T. (2015). Hemispheric asymmetry in cerebrovascular reactivity of the human primary motor cortex. *NMR in Biomedicine, 28,* 538–545.

Duman, E. A., & Canli, T. (2015). Influence of life stress, 5-HTTLPR genotype, and SLC6A4 methylation on gene expression and stress responses in healthy Caucasian males. *Biology of Mood and Anxiety Disorders, 5,* 2.

Dupierrix, E., de Boisferon, A. H., Meary, D., Lee, K., Quinn, P. C., Di Giorgio, E., et al. (2014). Preference for human eyes in human infants. *Journal of Experimental Child Psychology, 123,* 138–146.

Durschmid, S., Edwards, E., Reichert, C., Dewar, C., Hinrichs, H., Heinze, H. J., et al. (2016). Hierarchy of prediction errors for auditory events in human temporal and frontal cortex. *Proceedings of the National Academy of Sciences of the United States of America, 113*, 6755–6766.

Durschmid, S., Zaehle, T., Hinrichs, H., Heinze, H. J., Voges, J., Garrido, M. I., et al. (2016). Sensory deviancy detection measured directly within the human nucleus accumbens. *Cerebral Cortex, 26*, 1168–1175.

Earles, J. L., & Kersten, A. W. (2016). Why are verbs so hard to remember? *Cognitive Science, 23*. doi:10.1111/cogs.12374.

Ebisch, S. J., Ferri, F., & Gallese, V. (2014). Touching moments: desire modulates the neural anticipation of active romantic caress. *Frontiers in Behavioral Neuroscience*. doi:10.3389/frbeh.2014. 00060.

Eckstein, M., Scheele, D., Weber, K., Stoffel-Wagner, B., Maier, W., & Hurlemann, R. (2014). Oxytocin facilitates the sensation of social stress. *Human Brain Mapping, 35*, 4741–4750.

Edelman, R. T., & Baker, S. R. (2002). Self reported and actual physiological responses in social phobia. *British Journal of Clinical Psychology, 41*, 1–14.

Edwards, L. A., Wagner, J. B., Simon, C. E., & Hyde, D. C. (2016). Functional brain organization for number processing in pre-verbal infants. *Developmental Science, 19*, 757–769.

Eger, E. (2016). Neuronal foundations of human numerical representations. *Progress in Brain Research, 227*, 1–27.

Egidi, G., & Caramazza, A. (2016). Integration processes compared. *Journal of Cognitive Neuroscience, 28*, 1568–1583.

Eichenbaum, H. (2017). Memory: Organization and control. *Annual Review of Psychology, 68*, 1–20.

Einhauser, W., Rutishauser, U., & Koch, C. (2008). Task-demands can immediately reverse the effects of sensory-driven saliency in complex visual stimuli. *Journal of Vision, 8*, 1–19.

Eiseley, L. (1958). *Darwin's Century*. New York: Doubleday & Company.

Ekman, P. (1992). An argument for basic emotions. *Cognition and Emotion*, *6*, 169–200.

Ekman, P. (2016). What scientists who study emotion agree about. *Perspectives on Psychological Science*, *11*, 31–34.

El Karoui, I., King, J. R., Sitt, J., Meyniel, F., Van Gaal, S., Hasboun, D., et al. (2015). Event-related potential, time-frequency, and functional connectivity facets of local and global auditory novelty processing. *Cerebral Cortex*, *25*, 4203–4212.

El-Shamayleh, Y., & Pasupathy, A. (2016). Contour curvature as an invariant code for objects in visual area V4. *Journal of Neuroscience*, *36*, 5532–5543.

Ellis, A. (2016). *Men, Masculinities and Violence*. New York: Routledge.

Emberson, L. L., Richards, J. E., & Aslin, R. N. (2015). Top-down modulation in the infant brain. *Proceedings of the National Academy of Sciences of the United States of America*, *112*, 9585–9590.

Ennaceur, A., & Chazot, P. L. (2016). Preclinical animal anxiety research—Flaws and prejudices. *Pharmacology Research & Perspectives*, *4*, e00223.

Espy, K. A. (Ed.). (2016). The changing nature of executive control in preschool. *Monographs of the Society for Research in Child Development*, *81*, 7–150.

Evans, K. K., Haygood, T. M., Cooper, J., Culpan, A. M., & Wolfe, J. M. (2016). A half-second glimpse often lets radiologists identify breast cancer even when viewing the mammogram of the opposite breast. *Proceedings of the National Academy of Sciences of the United States of America*, *113*, 10252–10261.

Eysel, U. T. (2003). Illusions and perceived images in the primate brain. *Science*, *302*, 789–791.

Faasse, K., Martin, L. R., Grey, A., Gamble, G., & Petrie, K. J. (in press). Impact of brand or generic labeling on medication effectiveness and side effects. *Health Psychology*.

Fabbri, S., Stubbs, K. M., Cusack, R., & Culhan, J. C. (2016). Disentangling representations of object and grasp properties in the human brain. *Journal of Neuroscience, 36*, 7648–7662.

Farran, E. K., & Atkinson, L. (2016). The development of spatial category representation from 4 to 7 years. *British Journal of Developmental Psychology, 34*, 555–568.

Fedorenko, E., Scott, T. L., Brunner, P., Coon, W. G., Pritchett, B., Schalk, G., & Kanwisher, N. (2016). Neural correlates of the construction of sentence meaning. *Proceedings of the National Academy of Sciences of the United States of America, 113*, E6256–E6262.

Feinberg, T. E., & Mallatt, J. (2016). The nature of primary consciousness. *Consciousness and Cognition, 43*, 113–127.

Ferretti, A., Caulo, M., Del Gratta, C., Di Matteo, R., Merla, A., Montorsi, F., et al. (2005). Dynamics of male sexual arousal. *NeuroImage, 26*, 1086–1096.

Ferry, A. L., Hespos, S. I., & Waxman, S. R. (2010). Categorization in 3- and 4-month old infants. *Child Development, 81*, 472–479.

Fischer, C., Luaute, J., & Morlet, D. (2010). Event-related potentials (MMN and novelty P3) in permanent vegetative or minimally conscious states. *Clinical Neurophysiology, 121*, 1032–1042.

Fischer, J., Mikhael, J. G., & Kanwisher, N. (2016). Functional neuroanatomy of intuitive physical inference. *Proceedings of the National Academy of Sciences of the United States of America, 113*, E5012–E5081.

Fishell, G. (2016). Q & A. *Neuron, 91*, 725–727.

Floresco, S. B. (2015). The nucleus accumbens: An interface between cognition, emotion, and action. *Annual Review of Psychology, 66*, 25–62.

Flynn, K. A. (2008). In their own voices. *Journal of Child Sexual Abuse, 17*, 201–215.

Fochler, M., Felt, U., & Muller, R. (2016). Unsustainable growth, hypercompetition, and worth in life science research. *Minerva, 54*, 175–200.

Fontani, G., Farabollini, F., & Carli, G. (1984). Hippocampal electrical activity and behavior in the presence of novel environmental stimuli. *Behavioural Brain Research, 13*, 231–240.

Fonteyne, R., Vervliet, D., Hermans, D., Baeyens, F., & Vansteenwegen, D. (2009). Reducing chronic anxiety by making the threatening event predictable. *Behaviour Research and Therapy, 47*, 830–839.

Forkmann, T., Scherer, A., Meessen, J., Michal, M., Schachinger, H., Vogele, C., et al. (2016). Making sense of what you sense. *International Journal of Psychophysiology, 109*, 71–80.

Forss, S. I., Schuppli, C., Haiden, D., Zweifel, N., & van Schaik, C. P. (2015). Contrasting responses to novelty by wild and captive orang-utans. *American Journal of Primatology, 7*, 10. doi:10.1002/ajp.22445.

Fossat, P., Bacque-Cazenave, J., De Deurwaerdere, P., Delbecque, J. P., & Cattaert, D. (2014). Anxiety-like behavior in crayfish is controlled by serotonin. *Science, 344*, 1293–1297.

Fox, E., & Beevers, C. G. (2016). Differential sensitivity to the environment. *Molecular Psychiatry, 21*, 1657–1662.

Francis, R. C. (2015). *Domesticated*. New York: W. W. Norton.

Frantz, L. A. F., Schraiber, J. G., Madsen, O., Megens, M., Bosse, M., Paudel, Y., et al. (2015). Evidence of long-term gene flow and selection during domestication from analyses of Eurasian wild and domestic pig genomes. *Nature Genetics, 47*, 1141–1148.

Freed, D. M., & Corkin, S. (1988). Rate of forgetting in H. M. *Behavioral Neuroscience, 102*, 823–827.

Freiwald, W., Duchaine, D., & Yovel, G. (2016). Face processing systems. *Annual Review of Neuroscience, 39*, 325–346.

Frisell, T., Lichtenstein, P., & Langstrom, N. (2011). Violent crime in families. *Psychological Medicine, 41*, 97–105.

Fullana, M. A., Harrison, B. J., Soriano-Mas, C., Vervliet, B., Cardoner, N., Avila-Parcet, A., & Radua, J. (2016). Neural signatures of human fear conditioning. *Molecular Psychiatry, 21*, 500–508.

Furukawa, T. A., Cipriani, A., Atkinson, L. Z., Leucht, S., Ogawa, Y., Takeshima, N., et al. (2016). Placebo response rates in antidepressant trials. *Lancet. Psychiatry, 11*, 1059–1066.

Gagne, J. R., & Saudino, K. J. (2016). The development of inhibitory control in early childhood: A twin study from 2–3 years. *Developmental Psychology, 52*, 391–399.

Galison, P. (1997). *Image and logic.* Chicago, IL: University of Chicago Press.

Garces, P., Pereda, E., Hernandez-Tamames, J. A., Del-Pozo, F., Maestu, F., & Angel Pineda-Pardo, J. (2016). Multimodal description of whole brain connectivity: A comparison of resting state MEG, fMRI, and DWI. *Human Brain Mapping, 37*, 20–34.

Gardner, M. P., & Fontanini, A. (2014). Encoding and tracking of outcome-specific expectancy in the gustatory cortex of alert rats. *Journal of Neuroscience, 34*, 13000–13017.

Gates, K. M., & Molenaar, P. C. (2012). Group search algorithm recovers effective connectivity maps for individuals in homogeneous and heterogeneous samples. *NeuroImage, 63*, 310–319.

Genovesio, A., Seitz, L. K., Tsujimoto, S., & Wise, S. P. (2016). Context-dependent duration signals in the primate prefrontal cortex. *Cerebral Cortex, 26*, 3345–3356.

Gibbons, H., Schnuerch, R., & Stahl, J. (2016). From positivity to negativity bias. *Journal of Cognitive Neuroscience, 28*, 542–557.

Gibbons, M. B. C., Gallop, R., Thompson, D., Luther, D., Crits-Christoph, K., Jacobs, J., et al. (2016). Comparative effectiveness of cognitive therapy and dynamic psychotherapy for major depression disorder in a community mental health setting. *JAMA Psychiatry, 73*, 904–911.

Gilbert, C. (2012). Adult visual cortical plasticity. *Neuron, 75*, 9739–9746.

Gillan, C. M., & Daw, N. D. (2016). Taking psychiatry research on line. *Neuron, 91*, 19–23.

Gilron, R., Rosenblatt, J., Koyejo, O., Poldrack, R. A., & Mukamel, R. (2016). What's in a pattern? Examining the type of signal multivariate analysis uncovers at the group level. *NeuroImage, 146*, 113–120.

Gjorgjieva, J., Drion, G., & Marder, E. (2016). Computational implications of biophysical diversity and multiple timescales in neurons and synapses for circuit performance. *Current Opinion in Neurobiology, 37*, 44–52.

Gobbin, M. I., & Haxby, J. V. (2006). Neural response to the visual familiarity of faces. *Brain Research Bulletin, 71*, 76–82.

Godard, O., Baudouin, J. Y., Schaal, B., & Durand, K. (2016). Affective matching of odors and facial expressions in infants. *Developmental Science, 19*, 155–163.

Gonzalez-Garcia, N., Gonzalez, M. A., & Rendon, P. L. (2016). Neural activity related to discrimination and vocal production of consonant and dissonant musical intervals. *Brain Research*, Apr 28. pii:S0006–8993.

Gonzalez-Sulser, A., Parthier, D., Candela, A., McClure, C., Pastoll, H., Garden, D., et al. (2014). GABAergic projections from the medial septum selectively inhibit interneurons in the medial entorhinal cortex. *Journal of Neuroscience, 34*, 16739–16743.

Goodman, A., Heshmati, A., & Koupil, I. (2014). Family history of education predicts eating disorders across multiple generations among 2 million Swedish males and females. *PLoS One, 9*, e106475.doi:10.1371.

Goodman, J., Ressler, R. L., & Packard, M. G. (2016). The dorsolateral striatum selectively mediates extinction of habit memory. *Neurobiology of Learning and Memory, 136*, 54–62.

Goodnight, J. A., Donahue, K. L., Waldman, I. D., Van Hulle, C. A., Rathouz, P. J., Lahey, B. B., & D'Onofrio, B. M. (2016). Genetic and environmental contributions to associations between infant fussy temperament and antisocial behavior in childhood and adolescence. *Behavior Genetics, 46*, 680–692.

Graybiel, A. M. (2008). Habits, rituals, and the evaluative brain. *Annual Review of Neuroscience, 31*, 359–387.

Grayling, A. C. (2016). *The age of genius*. New York: Bloomsbury.

Greenhouse, I., Noah, S., Maddok, R. J., & Ivry, R. B. (2016). Individual differences in GABA content are reliable but are not uniform across the human cortex. *NeuroImage, 139,* 1–7.

Gregoire, M., Coll, M. P., Tremblay, M. P., Prkachin, K. M., & Jackson, P. L. (2016). Repeated exposure to others' pain reduces vicarious pain intensity estimation. *European Journal of Pain.* doi:10.1002/ ejp.888.

Gregory, S. W., & Webster, S. (1996). A nonverbal signal in voices of interview partners effectively predicts communication accommodation and social status perceptions. *Journal of Personality and Social Psychology, 70,* 1231–1240.

Gribbin, J. (2016). *13.8: The quest to find the true age of the universe and the theory of everything* . New Haven, CT: Yale University Press.

Grillon, C., Merikangas, K. R., Dierker, L., Snidman, N., Arriaga, R. I., Kagan, J., et al. (1999). Startle potentiation by threat of aversive stimuli and darkness in adolescents. *International Journal of Psychophysiology, 32,* 63–73.

Gross, J. J., & John, O. P. (2003). Individual differences in two emotion regulation processes: Implications for affect, relationships, and well-being. *Journal of Personality and Social Psychology, 85,* 348–362.

Haber, S. N. (2016). Corticostriatal circuitry. *Dialogues in Clinical Neuroscience, 18,* 7–22.

Haden, G. P., Nemeth, R., Torok, M., Dravucz, S., & Winkler, I. (2013). Context effects on processing widely deviant sounds in newborn infants. *Frontiers in Psychology, 4,* 674. doi:10.3389.

Hafed, Z. M., & Chen, C. Y. (2016). Sharper, stronger, faster upper visual field representation in primate superior colliculus. *Current Biology, 26,* 1647–1658.

Haith, M. M. (1998). Who put the cog in infant cognition? *Infant Behavior and Development, 21,* 167–179.

Hallock, H. L., Wang, A., & Griffin, A. L. (2016). Ventral midline thalamus is critical for hippocampal-prefrontal synchrony and spatial working memory. *Journal of Neuroscience, 36,* 8372–8389.

Hamel, A. F., Lutz, C. K., Coleman, K., Worlein, J. M., Peterson, E. J., Rosenberg, K. L., Novak, M. A., & Meyer, J. S. (2017). Responses to the human intruder test are related to hair cortisol phenotype and sex in rhesus macaques (*Macaca mulatta*). *American Journal of Primatology, 79,* 1–10.

Han, S., Northoff, G., Vogeley, K., Wexler, B. G., Kitayana, S., & Varnum, M. E. W. (2013). A critical neuroscience approach to the biological nature of the human brain. *Annual Review of Psychology, 64,* 335–359.

Handjaras, G., Ricciardi, E., Leo, A., Lenci, A., Cecchetti, L., Cosottini, M., et al. (2016). How concepts are encoded in the human brain. *Neuro-Image, 135,* 232–242.

Hanley, L. (2016). *Respectable.* London: Allen Lane.

Harvey, B. M., Klein, B. P., Petridou, N., & Dumoulin, S. O. (2013). Topographic representation of numerosity in the human parietal cortex. *Science, 341,* 1123–1126.

Hasselmo, M. E., & Stern, C. E. (2015). Current questions on space and time encoding. *Hippocampus, 25,* 744–752.

Hassett, J. M., Siebert, E. R., & Wallen, K. (2008). Sex differences in rhesus monkey toy preferences parallel those of children. *Hormones and Behavior, 54,* 359–364.

Haushofer, J., Baker, C. I., Livingstone, M. S., & Kanwisher, N. (2008). Privileged coding of convex shapes in human object-selective cortex. *Journal of Neurophysiology, 100,* 753–762.

Haworth-Hoeppner, S. (2017). *Family, culture, and self in the development of eating disorders.* New York: Routledge.

Haxby, J. V., Connolly, A. L., & Guntopalli, J. S. (2014). Decoding neural representational spaces using multivariate pattern analysis. *Annual Review of Neuroscience, 37,* 435–456.

Hayakawa, S., Costa, A., Foucart, A., & Keysar, B. (2016). Using a foreign language changes our choices. *Trends in Cognitive Sciences, 20,* 791–793.

He, B. J. (2013). Spontaneous and task-evoked brain activity negatively interact. *Journal of Neuroscience, 33,* 4672–4682.

He, L., Sillanpaa, M. J., Silventoinen, K., Kaprio, J., & Pitkaniemi, J. (2016). Estimating modifying effect of age on genetic and environmental variance components in twin models. *Genetics, 202,* 1313–1328.

Heaps, C., & Handel, S. (1999). Similarity and features of natural textures. *Journal of Experimental Psychology: Human Perception and Performance, 25,* 299–320.

Hebb, D. O. (1946). On the nature of fear. *Psychological Review, 53,* 259–276.

Hecht, E. E., Murphy, L. E., Gutman, D. A., Votaw, J. R., Schuster, D. M., Preuss, T. M., et al. (2013). Differences in neural activation for object-directed grasping in chimpanzees and humans. *Journal of Neuroscience, 33,* 14117–14134.

Hecht, E. E., Mahovetz, L. M., Preuss, T. M., & Hopkins, W. D. (2016). A neuroanatomical predictor of mirror self-recogntion in chimpanzees. *Social Cognitive and Affective Neuroscience.* doi:10.1093/scan/nsw159.

Hedger, N., Adams, W. J., & Garner, M. (2015). Fearful faces have a sensory advantage in the competition for awareness. *Journal of Experimental Psychology: Human Perception and Performance, 41,* 1748–1757.

Hedman, E., Axelssson, E., Andersson, E., Lekander, M., & Ljotsson, B. (2016). Experience-based cognitive-behavioral therapy via the internet and as bibliotherapy for somatic symptom disorder and illness anxiety disorder. *British Journal of Psychiatry, 209,* 407–413.

Hein, G., Morishima, Y., Leiberg, S., Sul, S., & Fehr, E. (2016). The brain's functional network architecture reveals human motives. *Science, 351,* 1074–1078.

Heir, T., Piatigorsky, A., & Weisath, L. (2009). Longitudinal changes in recalled life threat after a natural disaster. *British Journal of Psychiatry, 194,* 510–514.

Heisz, J. J., & Shedden, J. M. (2009). Semantic learning modifies perceptual face processing. *Journal of Cognitive Neuroscience, 21,* 1127–1134.

Henrich, J., Heine, S. J., & Norenzayan, A. (2010). The weirdest people in the world? *Behavioral and Brain Sciences, 33,* 61–83.

Henssen, A., Zilles, K., Palomero-Gallagher, N., Schleicher, A., Mohlberg, H., Gerboga, F., et al. (2016). Cytoarchitecture and probability maps of the human medial orbitofrontal cortex. *Cortex, 75,* 87–112.

Hepach, R., Haberl, K., Lambert, S., & Tomasello, M. (2017). Toddlers help anomymously. *Infancy, 22,* 130–145.

Herbener, E. S., Kagan, J., & Cohen, M. (1989). Shyness and olfactory threshold. *Personality and Individual Differences, 10,* 1159–1163.

Herdt, G. H. (1994). *Guardians of the flutes.* Chicago, IL: University of Chicago Press.

Hickok, G. (2014). *The myth of mirror neurons.* New York: W. W. Norton.

Hill, S. E., & Flom, R. (2007). 18- and 24-month-olds' discrimination of gender-consistent and inconsistent activities. *Infant Behavior and Development, 30,* 168–173.

Hiltzik, M. A. (2015). *Big science.* New York: Simon & Schuster.

Hirst, W., Phelps, E. A., Meksin, R., Vaidya, C. J., Johnson, M. K., Mitchell, K. J., et al. (2015). A ten-year follow-up of a study of memory for the attack of September 11, 2001. *Journal of Experimental Psychology. General, 144,* 604–623.

Hobson, N. M., & Inzlicht, M. (2016). The mere presence of an outgroup member disrupts the brain's feedback-monitoring system. *Social Cognitive and Affective Neuroscience, 11,* 1698–1706.

Hoffman, P., Lambon, R. M. A., & Rogers, T. T. (2013). Semantic diversity. *Behavior Research Methods, 45,* 718–730.

Hoge, C. W., Yehuda, R., Castro, C. A., McFarlane, A. C., Vermetten, E., Jetly, R., et al. (2016). Unintended consequences of changing the definition of Posttraumatic Stress Disorder in DSM-5. *JAMA Psychiatry, 73,* 750–752.

Holland, P. C., & Schiffino, F. L. (2016). Mini-review: Prediction errors, attention and associative learning. *Neurobiology of Learning and Memory, 131*, 207–215.

Holly, E. N., & Miczek, K. A. (2016). Ventral tegmental area dopamine revisited: Effects of acute and repeated stress. *Psychopharmacology, 233*, 163–186.

Holmes, A. J., Hollinshead, M. O., Roffman, J. L., Smoller, J. W., & Buckner, R. L. (2016). Individual differences in cognitive control circuit anatomy link sensation seeking, impulsivity, and substance use. *Journal of Neuroscience, 36*, 4038–4049.

Holstege, G., & Subramanian, H. H. (2016). Two different motor systems are needed to generate human speech. *Journal of Comparative Neurology, 524*, 1558–1577.

Holton, G. (2002). B. F. Skinner and P. W. Bridgman: The frustration of a Wahlverandschaft. In M. Heidelberger & F. Stadler (Eds.), *History of philosophy and science* (pp. 335–346). Dordrecht, the Netherlands: Kluwer.

Horner, A. J., Bisby, J. A., Wang, A., Bogus, K., & Burgess, N. (2016). The role of spatial boundaries in shaping long-term event representations. *Cognition, 154*, 151–164.

Horner, A. J., Bisby, J. A., Zotow, E., Bush, D., & Burgess, N. (2016). Gridlike processing of imagined navigation. *Current Biology, 26*, 842–847.

Howard, M. W., & Eichenbaum, H. (2015). Time and space in the hippocampus. *Brain Research, 1621*, 345–354.

Hsieh, J. C., Stone-Elander, S., & Ingvar, M. (1999). Anticipatory coping of pain expressed in the human anterior cingulate cortex. *Neuroscience Letters, 262*, 61–64.

Hubel, D. H., & Wiesel, T. N. (2005). *Brain and visual perception*. New York: Oxford University Press.

Huddleston, W. E., & DeYoe, E. A. (2008). The representation of spatial attention in human parietal cortex dynamically modulates with performance. *Cerebral Cortex, 18*, 1272–1280.

Huijgen, J., Dinkelacker, V., Lachat, F., Yahia-Cherif, L., El Karoui, I., Lemarechal, J. D., et al. (2015). Amygdala processing of social cues from faces. *Social Cognitive and Affective Neuroscience, 10,* 1568–1576.

Hull, C. L. (1943). *Principles of behavior.* New York: Appleton Century.

Husain, M., & Nachev, P. (2007). Space and the parietal cortex. *Trends in Cognitive Sciences, 11,* 30–36.

Hyman, S. E. (2016). Back to basics. *Nature Neuroscience, 19,* 1383–1388.

Iacovella, V., & Hasson, U. (2011). The relationship between BOLD signal and autonomic nervous system functions. *Magnetic Resonance Imaging, 29,* 1338–1345.

Ibos, G., & Freedman, D. J. (2016). Interaction between spatial and feature attention in posterior parietal cortex. *Neuron, 91,* 931–943.

Iijima, M., Arisaka, O., Minamoto, F., & Arai, Y. (2001). Sex differences in children's free drawings. *Hormones and Behavior, 40,* 99–104.

Immordino-Yang, M. H., Yang, X. F., & Damasio, H. (2014). Correlations between social-emotional feelings and anterior insula activity are independent from visceral states but influenced by culture. *Frontiers in Human Neuroscience, 8,* 728–736.

Infurna, F. J., & Luthar, S. S. (2016). Resilience to major life stresses is not as common as thought. *Perspectives on Psychological Science, 11,* 175–194.

Ingalhalikar, M., Smith, A., Parker, D., Satterthwaite, T. D., Elliott, M. A., Ruparel, K., et al. (2014). Sex differences in the structural connections of the human brain. *Proceedings of the National Academy of Sciences of the United States of America, 111,* 823–828.

Izquierdo, I., Furini, C. R., & Myskiw, J. C. (2016). Fear memory. *Physiological Reviews, 96,* 695–750.

Jaaskelainen, I. P., Pajula, J., Tohka, J., Lee, H. J., Kuo, W. J, & Lin, F. H. (2016). Brain hemodynamic activity during viewing and re-viewing of comedy movies explained by experienced humor. *Science Reports, 6,* 27741. doi:10.1038/srep27741.

Jackson, R. L., Hoffman, P., Pobric, G., & Lambon-Ralph, M. A. (2015). The nature and neural correlates of semantic association versus conceptual similarity. *Cerebral Cortex, 25,* 4319–4333.

Jaroszkieicz, G. (2016). *Images of time: Mind, science, and reality.* New York: Oxford University Press.

Jensen, K. B., Kaptchuk, T. J., Chen, X., Kirsch, I., Ingvar, M., Gollub, R. L., & Kong J. (2015). A neural mechanism for nonconscious activation of conditioned placebo and nocebo responses. *Cerebral Cortex, 25,* 3903–3910.

Jessen, S., & Grossmann, T. (2016). Neural and behavioral evidence for infants' sensitivity to the trustworthiness of faces. *Journal of Cognitive Neuroscience,* Jun 17. doi:10.1162/jocn_a 00999.

Jin, J., Zelano, C., Gottfried, J., & Mohanty, A. (2015). Human amygdala represents the complete spectrum of subjective valence. *Journal of Neuroscience, 35,* 15145–15156.

Jocham, G., Brodersen, K. H., Constantinescu, A. O., Kahn, M. C., Ianni, A. M., Walton, M. E., et al. (2016). Reward-guided learning with and without causal attribution. *Neuron, 90,* 177–190.

John, Y. J., Zikopoulos, B., Bullock, D., & Barbas, H. (2016). The emotional gatekeeper. *PLoS Computational Biology, 12,* e1004722.

Jonczyk, R., Boutonnet, B., Musial, K., Hoemann, K., & Thierry, G. (2016). The bilingual brain turns a blind eye to negative statements in the second language. *Cognitive, Affective & Behavioral Neuroscience, 16,* 527–540.

Jones, L. M., Fontanini, A., Sadacca, B. F., Miller, P., & Katz, D. B. (2007). Natural stimuli evoke dynamic sequences of states in sensory cortical ensembles. *Proceedings of the National Academy of Sciences of the United States of America, 104,* 18772–18777.

Jongkees, B. S., & Calzato, L. S. (2016). Spontaneous eye blink rate as a predictor of dopamine-related cognitive function—a review. *Neuroscience and Biobehavioral Reviews, 71,* 58–82.

Kadosh, R. C., Bahrami, B., Walsh. V., Butterworth, B., Popescu, T., & Price, C. J. (2011). Specialization in the human brain. *Frontiers in Human Neuroscience*, doi:org/10. 3389/fnhum.2011.

Kagan, J. (1970). The determinants of attention in the infant. *American Scientist*, *58*, 298–306.

Kagan, J. (1981). *The second year*. Cambridge, MA: Harvard University Press.

Kagan, J. (1994). *Galen's prophecy*. New York: Basic Books.

Kagan, J. (2008). In defense of qualitative changes in development. *Child Development*, *79*, 1606–1624.

Kagan, J. (2009). Categories of novelty and states of uncertainty. *Review of General Psychology*, *13*, 290–301.

Kagan, J., & Herschkowitz, N. (2005). *A young mind in a growing brain*. Mahwah, NJ: L. Erlbaum.

Kagan, J., Hosken, B., & Watson, S. (1961). Child's symbolic conceptualization of parents. *Child Development*, *32*, 625–636.

Kagan, J., Kearsley, R. B., & Zelazo, P. R. (1978). *Infancy*. Cambridge, MA: Harvard University Press.

Kagan, J., & Snidman, N. (2004). *The long shadow of temperament*. Cambridge, MA: Harvard University Press.

Kagan, J., Snidman, N., Kahn, V., & Towsley, S. (2007). The preservation of two infant temperaments into adolescence. *Monographs of the Society for Research in Child Development*, *72*, 1–75.

Kagan, J., Snidman, N., McManis, M., Woodward, S., & Hardway, C. (2002). One measure, one meaning: Multiple measures, clearer meaning. *Development and Psychopathology*, *14*, 463–475.

Kamali, A., Sair, H. I., Blitz, A. M., Riascos, R. F., Mirbagheri, S., Keser, Z., & Hasan, K. M. (2016). Revealing the ventral amygdalofugal pathway of the human limbic system using high spatial resolution diffusion tensor tractography. *Brain Structure & Function*.

Kamin, L. J. (1969). Predictability, surprise, attention and conditioning. In B. A. Campbell & R. M. Church (Eds.), *Punishment and aversive behavior* (pp. 279–296). New York: Appleton-Century-Crofts.

Kaminski, J., Call, J., & Fischer, J. (2004). Word learning in a domestic dog. *Science, 304,* 1682–1683.

Kamp, S. M., Potts, G. F., & Donchin, E. (2015). On the roles of distinctiveness and semantic expectancies in episodic encoding of emotional words. *Psychophysiology, 52,* 1599–1609.

Kanero, J., Hirsh-Pasek, K., & Golinkoff, R. M. (2016). Can a microwave heat up coffee? How English and Japanese-speaking children choose subjects in lexical causative sentences. *Journal of Child Language, 43,* 993–1019.

Kaplan, B. J. (2007). *Divided by faith.* Cambridge, MA: Harvard University Press.

Kaplan, K. A., Hirshman, J., Hernandez, A. R., Stefanick, M. L., Hoffman, A. R., Redline, S., et al. (2016). When a gold standard isn't so golden. *Biological Psychology, 123,* 37–46.

Kaplan, R. L., Levine, L. J., Lench, H. C., & Safer, M. A. (2016). Forgetting feelings. *Emotion, 16,* 309–319.

Kaplan, Z., Matar, M. A., Kamin, R., Sadan, T., & Cohen, H. (2005). Stress-related responses after 3 years of exposure to terror in Israel. *Journal of Clinical Psychiatry, 66,* 1146–1154.

Kashdan, T. B., & Farmer, A. S. (2014). Differentiating emotions across contexts. *Emotion, 14,* 619–631.

Kawabata, H., & Zeki, S. (2004). Neural correlates of beauty. *Journal of Neurophysiology, 91,* 1699–1705.

Kayal, M., Widen, S., & Russell, J. A. (2015). Context is more powerful than we think. *Emotion, 15,* 287–291.

Keating, C., & Keating, E. C. (1993). Monkeys and mug shots. *Journal of Comparative Psychology, 107,* 131–139.

Keesee, N. J., Currier, J. M., & Neimeyer, R. A. (2008). Predictors of grief following the death of one's child: The contribution of finding meaning. *Journal of Clinical Psychology, 64*, 1145–1163.

Kendler, K. S. (2016). The phenomenology of major depression and the representativeness and nature of DSM criteria. *American Journal of Psychiatry, 173*, 771–780.

Kennedy, T. M., & Ceballo, R. (2016). Emotionally numb. *Developmental Psychology, 52*, 778–789.

Key, A. P., Jones, D., & Peters, S. U. (2016). Response to own name in children. *Biological Psychology, 119*, 210–215.

Kim, H. J., Yoon, D. Y., Kim, E. S., Lee, K., Bae, J. S., & Lee, J. H. (2016). The 100 most cited articles in neuroimaging. *NeuroImage, 139*, 149–156.

Kim, J. H., & Ress, D. (2016). Arterial impulse model for the BOLD response to brief neural activation. *NeuroImage, 124*, Part A, 394–408.

Kim, N. Y., & McCarthy, G. (2016). Task influences pattern discriminability for faces and bodies in ventral occipitotemporal cortex. *Social Neuroscience, 27*, 1–10.

Kim, T., & Freeman, R. D. (2016). Direction selectivity of neurons in the visual cortex is non-linear and lamina-dependent. *European Journal of Neuroscience, 43*, 1389–1399.

Kim, M. J., Solomon, K. M., Neta, M., Davis, C., Oler, J. A., Mazzulla, E. C., et al. (2016). A face versus non-face context influences amygdala responses to masked fearful eye whites. *Social Cognitive and Affective Neuroscience, 11*, 1933–1941.

Kimble, C. E., & Seidel, S. D. (1991). Vocal signs of confidence. *Journal of Nonverbal Behavior, 15*, 99–105.

Kitanaka, J. (2012). *Depression in Japan*. Princeton, NJ: Princeton University Press.

Kleint, N. I., Wittchen, H. U., & Lueken, U. (2015). Probing the interoceptive network by listening to heartbeats: An fMRI study. *PLoS One, 10*, e0133164. doi:10.1377.

Koch, C., Massimini, M., Boly, M., & Tononi, G. (2016). Neural correlates of consciousness. *Nature Reviews. Neuroscience, 17,* 307–321.

Koh, M. T., Wilkins, E. E., & Bernstein, I. L. (2003). Novel tastes elevate c-fos expression in the central amygdala and insular cortex. *Behavioral Neuroscience, 117,* 1416–1422.

Kohn, A., Coen-Cagli, R., Kanitscheider, I., & Pouget, A. (2016). Correlations and neuronal population information. *Annual Review of Neuroscience, 39,* 233–256.

Koops, K., Furuichi, T., Hashimoto, C., & van Schaik, C. P. (2015). Sex differences in object manipulation in wild immature chimpanzees (*Pan troglodytes schweinfurthii*) and bonobos (*Pan paniscus*). *PLoS One, 10,* e0139909. doi:10.1377.

Koppel, J., & Rubin, D. C. (2016). Recent advances in understanding the reminiscence bump. *Current Directions in Psychological Science, 25,* 135–140.

Koppensteiner, M., Stephan, P., & Jaschke, J. P. (2016). Shaking takete and flowing maluma. Non-sense words are associated with motion patterns. *PLoS One, 11,* e0150610.

Korte, M., & Schmitz, D. (2016). Cellular and system biology of memory. *Physiological Reviews, 96,* 647–693.

Koscik, T., O'Leary, D., Moser, D. J., Andreassen, N. C., & Nopoulos, P. (2009). Sex differences in parietal lobe morphology. *Brain and Cognition, 69,* 451–459.

Koster, B., Sondergaard, J., Nielsen, J. B., Allen, M., Olsen, A., & Bentzen, J. (2016). The validated sun exposure questionnaire. *British Journal of Dermatology, 14.* doi:10.1111/bjd.14861.

Koster, R., Seow, T. X., Dolan, R. J., & Duzel, E. (2016). Stimulus novelty energizes actions in the absence of explicit reward. *PLoS One, 11*(7), e0159120. doi:10.137/journal.pone.0159120.

Kottler, J. (2010). *The assassin and the therapist.* New York: Routledge.

Kraemer, H. C. (2015). A source of false findings in published research studies: Adjusting for covariates. *JAMA Psychiatry*, *72*, 961–962.

Kremkow, J., Jin, J., Wang, Y., & Alonso, J. M. (2016). Principles underlying sensory map topography in primary visual cortex. *Nature*, *533*, 52–57.

Kret, M. E., Jaasma, L., Bionda, T., & Wijnen, J. G. (2016). Bonobos (*Pan paniscus*) show an attentional bias toward conspecifics' emotions. *Proceedings of the National Academy of Sciences of the United States of America*, *113*, 3761–3766.

Kristensen, S., Garcea, F. E., Mahon, B. Z., & Almeida, J. (2016). Temporal frequency tuning reveals interaction between the dorsal and ventral visual streams. *Journal of Cognitive Neuroscience*, Apr 15. doi:10.1162/jocn_a_00969.

Kruger, T., Fiedler, K., Koch, A. S., & Alves, H. (2014). Response category width as a psychophysical manifestation of construal level and distance. *Personality and Social Psychology Bulletin*, *40*, 501–512.

Krupenye, C., Kano, F., Hirata, S., Call, J., & Tomasello, M. (2016). Great apes anticipate that other individuals will act according to false beliefs. *Science*, *354*, 110–114.

Krys, K., Vauclair, C.-M., Capaldi, C. A., Lun, V. M., Bond, M. H., Domínguez-Espinosa, A., et al. (2016). Be careful where you smile. *Journal of Nonverbal Behavior*, *40*, 101–116.

Kufahl, P., Li, Z., Risinger, R., Rainey, C., Piacentine, L., Wu, G., et al. (2008). Expectation modulates human brain responses to acute cocaine. *Biological Psychiatry*, *63*, 222–230.

Kuhn, G., & Rensink, R. A. (2016). The vanishing ball illusion. *Cognition*, *148*, 64–70.

Kumaran, D., & Maguire, E. A. (2007). Match-mismatch processes underlie human hippocampal responses to associative novelty. *Journal of Neuroscience*, *27*, 8517–8524.

Kunecke, J., Sommer, W., Schacht, A., & Palazova, M. (2015). Embodied simulation of emotional valence. *Psychophysiology*, *52*, 1590–1598.

Kuwabara, M., & Smith, L. B. (2016). Cultural differences in visual object recognition in 3-year-old children. *Journal of Experimental Child Psychology*, *147*, 22–38.

Kwan, V. S., Wojcik, S. P., Miron-Shatz, T., Votruba, A. M., & Olivola, C. Y. (2012). Effects of symptom presentation on perceived disease risk. *Psychological Science*, *23*, 381–385.

Labrenz, F., Icenhour, A., Schlamann, M., Forsting, M., Bingel, U., & Elsenbruch, S. (2016). From Pavlov to pain: How predictability affects the anticipation and processing of visceral pain in a fear conditioning paradigm. *NeuroImage*, *130*, 104–114.

Lahey, B. B., Lee, S. S., Sibley, B. H., Applegate, B., Molina, B. S. G., & Pelham, W. B. (2016). Predictors of adolescent outcomes among 4–6-year-old-children with attention-deficit/hyperactivity disorder. *Journal of Abnormal Psychology*, *125*, 168–181.

Lahti, J., Raikkonen, K., Ekelund, J., Peltonen, L., Raitakari, O. T., & Keltikangas-Jarvinen, L. (2006). Socio-demographic characteristics moderate the association between DRD4 and novelty seeking. *Personality and Individual Differences*, *40*, 533–543.

Landry, G. J., Best, J. R., & Liu-Ambrose, T. (2015). Measuring sleep quality in older adults. *Frontiers in Aging Neuroscience*, *7*, 166. doi:10.338.

Langs, G., Wang, D., Golland, P., Mueller, S., Pan, R., Sabuncu, M. R., et al. (2016). Identifying shared brain networks in individuals by decoupling functional and anatomic variability. *Cerebral Cortex*, *26*, 4004–4014.

Lankinen, K., Smeds, E., Tikka, P., Pihko, E., Hari, R., & Koskinen, M. (2016). Haptic contents of a movie dynamically engage the spectator's sensorimotor cortex. *Human Brain Mapping*, *37*, 4061–4068.

Lanza, S. T., & Cooper, B. R. (2016). Latent class analysis for developmental research. *Child Development Perspectives*, *10*, 59–64.

Lavan, N., Scott, S. K., & McGettigan, C. (2016). Laugh like you mean it: Authenticity modulates acoustic, physiological and perceptual properties of laughter. *Journal of Nonverbal Behavior, 40*, 133–149.

Lavigne, J. V., Gouze, K. R., Hopkins, J., & Bryant, F. B. (2016). Multi-domain predictions of Attention Deficit/Hyperactivity disorder symptoms in preschool children. *Child Psychiatry and Human Development, 47*, 841–856.

Learmonth, A. E., Newcombe, N. S., & Huttenlocher, J. (2001). Toddlers' use of metric information and landmarks to reorient. *Journal of Experimental Child Psychology, 80*, 225–244.

Le Doux, J. E. (2014). Coming to terms with fear. *Proceedings of the National Academy of Sciences of the United States of America, 111*, 2871–2878.

Le Doux, J. E., & Pine, D. S. (2016). Using neuroscience to help understand fear and anxiety:A two-system framework. *American Journal of Psychiatry, 173*, 1083–1093.

Le Doux, J. E., Miscarello, J., Sears, R., & Campese, V. (2016). The birth, death and resurrection of avoidance. *Molecular Psychiatry, 22*, 24–36.

Lee, B. X., Marotta, P. L., Blay-Tofey, M., Wang, W., & de Bourmant, S. (2014). Economic correlates of violent death rates in forty countries, 1962–2008. *Aggression and Violent Behavior, 19*, 729–737.

Lee, E., Kang, J. I., Park, I. H., Kim, J. J., & An, S. K. (2008). Is a neutral face really evaluated as being emotionally neutral? *Psychiatry Research, 157*, 77–85.

Lee, K. H., & Siegle, G. J. (2014). Different brain activity in response to emotional faces alone and augmented by contextual information. *Psychophysiology, 51*, 1147–1157.

LeFevre, J. A. (2016). Numerical cognition: Adding it up. *Canadian Journal of Experimental Psychology, 70*, 2–11.

Lefkowitz, E. S., Vasilenko, S. A., & Leavitt, C. E. (2016). Oral vs. vaginal sex experiences and consequences among first-year college students. *Archives of Sexual Behavior, 45*, 329–337.

Leibovich, T., & Henik, A. (2014). Comparing performance in discrete and continuous comparison tasks. *Quarterly Journal of Experimental Psychology, 67*, 1–19.

Lents, N. H. (2016). *Not so different.* New York: Columbia University Press.

Leonhardt, D. (2013). In climbing the income ladder, location matters. *New York Times*, July 22.

Lescroart, M. D., Stansbury, D. E., & Gallant, J. L. (2015). Fourier power, subjective distance, and object categories all provide plausible models of BOLD responses in scene-selective visual areas. *Frontiers in Computational Neuroscience, 9*, 135. doi:10.3309.

Li, K., Nakajima, M., Ibanez-Tallon, I., & Heintz, N. (2016). A cortical circuit for sexually dimorphic oxytocin-dependent anxiety behaviors. *Cell, 167*, 60–72.

Libet, B., Gleason, C. A., Wright, E. W., & Pearl, D. K. (1983). Time of conscious intention to act in relation to onset of cerebral activity (readiness-potential). *Brain, 106*, 623–642.

Lin, C. S., Hsieh, J. C., Yeh, T. C., Lee, S. Y., & Niddam, D. M. (2013). Functional dissociation within insular cortex. *Brain Research, 1493*, 40–47.

Logothetis, N. K. (2014). Neural-event-triggered FMRI of large-scale neural networks. *Current Opinion in Neurobiology, 31*, 214–222.

Love, J. M., Chazan-Cohen, R., Raikes, H., & Brooks-Gunn, J. (2013). What makes a difference: Early Head Start evaluation findings in a developmental context. *Monographs of the Society for Research in Child Development, 78*, 1–172.

Luecken, L. J., & Roubinow, D. S. (2012). Pathways to lifespan health following childhood parental death. *Social and Personality Psychology Compass, 6*, 243–257.

Luke, N., & Banerjee, R. (2013). Differential associations between childhood maltreatment experiences and social understanding. *Developmental Review, 33*, 1–28.

Luo, Q., Holroyd, T., Jones, M., Hendler, T., & Blair, J. (2007). Neural dynamics for facial threat processing as revealed by gamma band synchronization using MEG. *NeuroImage, 34*, 839–847.

Lupyan, G., & Dale, R. (2016). Why are there different languages? *Trends in Cognitive Sciences, 20*, 649–660.

Ma, L., Hyman, J. M., Durstewitz, D., Phillips, A. G., & Seamans, J. K. (2016). A quantitative analysis of context-dependent remapping of medial frontal cortex neurons and ensembles. *Journal of Neuroscience, 36*, 8258–8272.

MacDonald, M. P. (1999). *All souls*. Boston, MA: Beacon Press.

Macefield, V. G., & Henderson, L. A. (2016). Real-time imagery of cortical and subcortical sites of cardiovascular control. *Journal of Neurophysiology, 116*, 1199–1207.

Madore, K. P., Szpunar, K. K., Addis, D. R., & Schacter, D. L. (2016). Episodic specificity induction impacts activity in a core brain network during construction of imagined future experiences. *Proceedings of the National Academy of Sciences of the United States of America, 113*, 10696–10701.

Maes, E., Boddez, Y., Alfei, J. M., Kryptos, A. M., D'Hooge, R., De Houwer, J., & Beckers (2016). The elusive nature of the blocking effect. *Journal of Experimental Psychology. General, 145*, e49–e71.

Maitre, J. L., Tuilier, H., Illukkumbura, R., Eismann, B., Niwayama, R., Nedelec, F., et al. (2016). Asymmetric division of contractile domains couples cell position and fate specification. *Nature, 536*, 344–348.

Manuck, S. B., Flory, J. D., Ferrell, R. F., & Muldoon, M. F. (2004). Socioeconomic status covaries with central nervous system serotonergic responsivity as a function of allelic variation in the serotonin transporter gene–linked polymorphic region. *Psychoneuroendocrinology, 29*, 651–668.

Marder, E. (2015). Understanding brains. *PLoS Biology, 13*, e1002147.

Marder, E. (2016). Computational implications of biophysical diversity and multiple timescales in neurons and synapses for circuit performance. *Current Opinion in Neurobiology, 37,* 44–52.

Marder, E., Gutierrez, G., & Nusbaum, M. P. (2016). Complicating connectomes: Electrical coupling creates parallel pathways and degenerate circuit mechanisms. *Developmental Neurobiology,* Jun 17. doi:10.1002/dneu.22410.

Mason, R. A., & Just, M. A. (2016). Neural representations of physics concepts. *Psychological Science,* Apr 25. pii:095679761661941.

Matsubayashi, T., Sawada, Y., & Ueda, M. (2014). Does the installation of blue lights on train platforms shift suicide to another installation? *Journal of Affective Disorders, 169,* 57–60.

Matsuhashi, M., & Hallett, M. (2008). The timing of the conscious intention to move. *European Journal of Neuroscience, 28,* 2344–2355.

Maurer, D., Pathman, T., & Mondloch, C. J. (2006). The shape of boubas. *Developmental Science, 9,* 316–322.

Mayer, A., Schwiedrzik, C. M., Wibral, M., Singer, W., & Melloni, L. (2016). Expecting to see a letter: Alpha oscillations as carriers of top-down sensory predictions. *Cerebral Cortex, 26,* 3146–3160.

McCarthy, M. M. (2011). A lumpers versus splitters approach to sexual differentiation of the brain. *Frontiers in Neuroendocrinology, 32,* 114–123.

McCarthy-Jones, S. (2012). *Hearing voices.* New York: Cambridge University Press.

McCutcheon, J. E., Conrad, K. L., Carr, S. B., Ford, K. A., McGehee, D. S., & Marinelli, M. (2012). Dopamine neurons in the ventral tegmental area fire faster in adolescent rats than in adults. *Journal of Neurophysiology, 108,* 1620–1630.

McGarry, L. M., & Carter, A. G. (2016). Inhibitory gating of basolateral amygdala inputs to the prefrontal cortex. *Journal of Neuroscience, 36,* 9391–9406.

McGinn, C. (2002). *The making of a philosopher.* New York: HarperCollins.

McHugh, S. B., Barkus, C., Huber, A., Capitao, L., Lima, J., Lowry, J. P., & Bannerman, D. M. (2014). Aversive prediction error signals in the human amygdala. *Journal of Neuroscience, 34,* 9024–9033.

McLeod, G. F. H., Horwood, L. J., & Fergusson, D. M. (2016). Adolescent depression, adult mental health and psychosocial outcomes at 30 and 35 years. *Psychological Medicine, 46,* 1401–1412.

Mehu, M., & Scherer, K. R. (2015). Emotion categories and dimensions in the facial communication of affect: An integrated approach. *Emotion, 15,* 798–811.

Meijer, E. H., Verschuere, B., Gamer, M., Merckelbach, H., & Ben-Shakhar, G. (2016). Deception detection with behavioral, autonomic, and neural measures. *Psychophysiology, 53,* 593–604.

Mellor, D. H. (Ed.). (1990). *F. P. Ramsey: Philosophical papers.* New York: Cambridge University Press.

Mendes, W. B., Blascovich, J., Hunter, S. B., Lickel, B., & Jost, J. T. (2007). Threatened by the unexpected. *Journal of Personality and Social Psychology, 92,* 698–716.

Mesquita, L. T., Abreu, A. R., de Abreu, A. R., de Souza, A. A., de Noronha, S. R., Silva, F. C., Campos, G. S., Chianca, D. A., Jr., & de Menezes, R. C. (2016). New insights on amygdala: Basomedial amygdala regulates the physiological response to social novelty. *Neuroscience,* May 31. pii:S0306–4522(16) 30212–3.

Metusalem, R., Kutas, M., Urbach, T. P., & Elman, J. L. (2016). Hemispheric asymmetry in event knowledge activation during incremental language comprehension. *Neuropsychologia,* Feb 12. pii:S0028–3932.

Meyer, A., Lerner, M. D., De LosReyes, A., Laird, R. D., & Hajcak, G. (2017). Considering ERP difference scores as individual difference measures: Issues with subtraction and alternative approaches. *Psychophysiology, 54,* 114–122.

Meyerhoff, J., & Rohan, K. J. (2016). Treatment expectations for cognitive-behavioral therapy and light therapy for seasonal affective disorder. *Journal of Consulting and Clinical Psychology, 84*, 898–906.

Michalczyk, L., Millard, A. L., Martin, O. Y., Lumley, A. J., Emerson, B. C., Chapman, T., & Gage, M. J. (2011). Inbreeding promotes female promiscuity. *Science, 333*, 1739–1742.

Mik, A., Realo, A., & Allik, J. (2015). Retrospective ratings of emotions. *Frontiers in Psychology, 6*, 2020.

Milaniak, I., & Widom, C. S. (2015). Does child abuse and neglect increase risk for perpetration of violence inside and outside the home? *Psychology of Violence, 5*, 246–255.

Milgram, S. (1974). *Obedience to authority.* New York: Harper & Row.

Miller, C. J., Newcorn, J. H., & Halperin, J. M. (2010). Fading memories. *Journal of Attention Disorders, 14*, 7–14.

Miller, G. E., Cohen, S., Janicki-Deverts, D., Brody, G. H., & Chen, E. (2016). Viral challenge reveals further evidence of skin-deep resilience in African Americans from disadvantaged backgrounds. *Health Psychology, 35*, 1225–1234.

Miller, G. E., Murphy, M. L., Cashman, R., Ma, R., Ma, J., & Cole, S. W. (2014). Greater inflammatory activity and blunted glucocorticoid signaling in monocytes of chronically stressed caregivers. *Brain, Behavior, and Immunity, 41*, 191–199.

Miller, K. J., Hermes, D., Witthoft, N., Rao, R. P., & Ojemann, J. G. (2015). The physiology of perception in human temporal lobe is specialized for contextual novelty. *Journal of Neurophysiology, 114*, 250–263.

Miller, M. B., Donovan, C. L., Van Horn, J. D., German, E., Sokol-Hessner, P., & Wolford, G. L. (2009). Unique and persistent individual patterns of brain activity across different memory retrieval tasks. *NeuroImage, 48*, 625–635.

Miller, R., Stalder, T., Jarczok, M., Almeida, P. M., Badrick, E., Bartels, M., et al. (2016). The CIRCORT database. *Psychoneuroendocrinology*, *73*, 16–23.

Miozzo, M., & Laeng, B. (2016). Why Saturday could be both green and red in synesthesia. *Cognitive Processing*, *17*(4), 337–355.

Mitchell, A. S. (2015). The mediodorsal thalamus as higher order thalamus relay nucleus important for learning and decision. *Neuroscience and Biobehavioral Reviews*, *54*, 57–79.

Mix, K. S., Levine, S. C., & Newcombe, N. S. (2016). Development of quantitative thinking across correlated dimensions. In A. Henik (Ed.), *Continuous issues in numerical cognition* (pp. 3–35). New York: Elsevier.

Mobbs, D., Yu, R., Meyer, M., Passamonti, L., Seymour, B., Calder, A. J., et al. (2009). A key role for similarity in vicarious reward. *Science*, *324*, 900.

Moffitt, T. E., Houts, R., Asherson, P., Belsky, D. W., Corcoran, D. L., Hammerle, M., et al. (2015). Is adult ADHD a childhood-onset neurodevelopmental disorder? Evidence from a four-decade longitudinal cohort study. *American Journal of Psychiatry*, *172*, 967–977.

Montes-Lourido, P., Bermudez, M. A., Romero, M. C., & Vicente, A. F. (2016). Spatial frequency components of images modulate neural activity in monkey amygdala. *Perception*, *45*, 375–385.

Moore, R., Call, J., & Tomasello, M. (2015). Production and comprehension of gestures between orang-utans (*Pongo pygmaeus*) in a referential communication game. *PloS One*, e0129726. doi:10.13771.

Morel, S., Beaucousin, V., Perrin, M., & George, N. (2012). Very early modulation of brain responses to neutral faces by a single prior association with an emotional context. *NeuroImage*, *16*, 1461–1470.

Morris, A. P., Bremmer, F., & Krekelberg, B. (2016). The dorsal visual system predicts future and remembers past eye position. *Frontiers in Systems Neuroscience*, *10*, 9. doi:10.3389.

Mosher, C. P., Zimmerman, P. E., & Gothard, K. M. (2014). Neurons in the monkey amygdala detect eye-contact during naturalistic social interaction. *Current Biology, 24,* 2459–2464.

Mourao, F. A. G., Lockmann, A. L. V., Castro, G. P., Medeiros, D. C., Reis, M. P., Pereira, G. S., et al. (2016). Triggering different brain states using asynchronous serial communication to the rat amygdala. *Cerebral Cortex, 26,* 1866–1877.

Muehlhan, M., Kirschbaum, C., Wittchen, H. U., & Alexander, N. (2015). Epigenetic variation in the serotonin transporter gene predicts resting state functional connectivity strength within the salience-network. *Human Brain Mapping, 36,* 4361–4371.

Mur, M., Ruff, D. A., Bodurka, J., Bandettini, P. A., & Kriegeskorte, N. (2010). Face-identity change activation outside the face system. *Cerebral Cortex, 20,* 2027–2042.

Muri, R. M. (2016). Cortical control of facial expression. *Journal of Comparative Neurology, 524,* 1578–1585.

Musliner, K. L., Munk-Olsen, T., Laursen, T. M., Eaton, W. W., Zandi, P. P., & Mortensen, P. B. (2016). Heterogeneity in 10-year course trajectories of moderate to severe major depression. *JAMA Psychiatry, 73,* 346–353.

Nakano, T., Kato, M., Morito, Y., Itoi, S., & Kitazawa, S. (2013). Blink-related momentary activation of the default mode network while viewing videos. *Proceedings of the National Academy of Sciences of the United States of America, 110,* 702–706.

Namburi, P., Al-Hasani, R., Calhoon, G. G., Bruchas, M. R., & Tye, K. M. (2016). Architectural representation of valence in the limbic system. *Neuropsychopharmacology, 41,* 1697–1715.

Namdar, G., Ganel, T., & Algon, D. (2016). The extreme relativity of perception. *Journal of Experimental Psychology. General, 145,* 509–515.

Napadow, V., Li, A., Loggia, M. L., Kim, J., Mawla, I., Desbordes, G., et al. (2015). The imagined itch: Brain circuitry supporting nocebo-induced itch in atopic dermatitis patients. *Allergy, 70,* 1485–1492.

Nasr, S., Echavarria, C. E., & Tootell, R. B. H. (2014). Thinking outside the box. *Journal of Neuroscience, 34*, 6721–6735.

Nelson, C. A., Fox, N. A., & Zeanah, C. H. (2014). *Romania's abandoned children*. Cambridge, MA: Harvard University Press.

Nestor, A., Plaut, D. C., & Behrmann, M. (2016). Feature-based face representations and image reconstruction from behavioral and neural data. *Proceedings of the National Academy of Sciences of the United States of America, 113*, 416–421.

Nieh, E. H., Vander Wheele, C. M., Matthews, G. A., Presbrey, K. N., Wichman, R., Leppla, C. A., et al. (2016). Inhibitory input from the lateral hypothalamus to the ventral tegmental area disinhibits dopamine neurons and promotes behavioral activation. *Neuron, 90*, 1286–1298.

Nisbett, R. E. (2015). *Mindware*. New York: Farrar, Straus & Giroux.

Nisbett, R. E., Peng, K., Choi, I., & Norenzayan, A. (2001). Culture and systems of thought. *Psychological Review, 108*, 291–310.

Nishijo, H., Ono, T., & Nishino, H. (1988). Topographic distribution of modality-specific amygdalar neurons in alert monkey. *Journal of Neuroscience, 8*, 3556–3569.

Nishith, P., Nixon, R. D. V., & Resick, P. A. (2005). Resolution of trauma-related guilt following treatment of PTSD in female rape victims. *Journal of Affective Disorders, 86*, 259–265.

Nobes, G., Panagiotaki, G., & Bartholomew, K. J. (2016). The influence of intention, outcome and question-wording on children's and adult's moral judgments. *Cognition, 157*, 190–204.

Nobile, M., Giorda, R., Marino, C., Carlet, O., Pastore, V., Vanzin, L., et al. (2007). Socioeconomic status mediates the genetic contribution of the dopamine receptor D4 and serotonin transporter linked promoter region repeat polymorphisms to externalization in preadolescents. *Development and Psychopathology, 19*, 1147–1160.

Nolan, E., & Kagan, J. (1978). Psychological factors in the face-hands test. *Archives of Neurology, 35*, 41–42.

Nordenskjold, A., Martensson, B., Pettersson, A., Heintz, E., & Landen, M. (2016). Effects of Hesel-coil deep transcranial magnetic stimulation for depression—A systematic review. *Nordic Journal of Psychiatry, 19*, 1–6.

Nunez, P. L., & Srinivasan, R. (2007). Hearts don't love and brains don't pump. *Journal of Consciousness Studies, 14*, 20–34.

Odegaard, B., & Shams, L. (2016). The brain's tendency to bind audiovisual signals is stable but not general. *Psychological Science, 27*, 583–591.

Offer, D., Kaiz, M., Howard, K. I., & Bennettt, E. S. (2000). The altering of reported experiences. *Journal of the American Academy of Child and Adolescent Psychiatry, 39*, 735–742.

Ogden, C. K. (1967). *Opposition*. Bloomington: Indiana University Press.

Oler, J. A., Tromp, D. P., Fox, A. S., Kovner, R., Davidson, R. J., Alexander, A. L., et al. (2016). Connectivity between the central nucleus of the amygdala and the bed nucleus of the stria terminalis in the non-human primate. *Brain Structure & Function*, doi:10.1007/s00429-016-1198-9.

Olkowicz, S., Kocourek, M., Lucan, R. K., Portes, M., Fitch, W. T., Herculano-Houzel, S., & Nemec, P. (2016). Birds have primate-like numbers of neurons in the forebrain. *Proceedings of the National Academy of Sciences of the United States of America, 113*, 7255–7260.

Ortuno, T., Grieve, K. L., Cao, R., Cudeiro, J., & Rivadulla, C. (2014). Bursting thalamic responses in awake monkey contribute to visual detection and are modulated by corticofugal feedback. *Frontiers in Behavioral Neuroscience, 8*, 198.

Osgood, C. E., Suci, G. J., & Tannenbaum, P. H. (1957). *The measurement of meaning*. Urbana: University of Illinois Press.

Oswald, J. A., & Wu, S. (2010). Objective confirmation of subjective measures of human well-being. *Science, 327*, 576–579.

Otto, H., & Keller, H. (Eds.). (2014). *Different faces of attachment*. New York: Cambridge University Press.

Over, H., Vaish, A., & Tomasello, M. (2016). Do young children accept responsibility for negative actions of ingroup members? *Cognitive Development*, *40*, 24–32.

Owen, A. M., Coleman, M. R., Boly, M., Davis, M. H., Laureys, S., & Pickard, J. D. (2006). Detecting awareness in the vegetative state. *Science*, *313*, 1402.

Owens, A. P., Low, D. A., Iodice, V., Critchley, H. D., & Mathias, C. J. (2016). The genesis and presentation of anxiety in disorders of autonomic over excitation. *Autonomic Neuroscience*, pii: S1566-0702 (16)30225-9.

Palombo, D. J., Keane, M. M., & Verfaellie, M. (2016). Does the hippocampus keep track of time? *Hippocampus*, *26*, 372–379.

Paolacci, G., & Chandler, J. (2014). Inside the Turk: Understanding Mechanical Turk as a participant pool. *Current Directions in Psychological Science*, *23*, 184–188.

Pape, H. C. (2005). GABAergic neurons: Gate masters of the amygdala, mastered by dopamine. *Neuron*, *48*, 877–879.

Park, H. D., Bernasconi, F., Bello-Ruiz, J., Pfeiffer, C., Salomon, R., & Blanke, O. (2016). Transient modulations of neural responses to heartbeats covary with bodily self-consciousness. *Journal of Neuroscience*, *36*, 8453–8460.

Park, S., Lee, J. M., Kim, J. W., Cho, D. Y., Yun, H. J., Han, D. H., et al. (2015). Associations between serotonin transporter gene (SLC6A4) methylation and clinical characteristics and cortical thickness in children with ADHD. *Psychological Medicine*, *45*, 3009–3017.

Parkes, L., Perry, C., & Goodin, P. (2016). Examining the N400 in affectively negative sentences. *Psychophysiology*, *53*, 689–704.

Parkinson, J., & Haggard, P. (2015). Choosing to stop: Responses evoked by externally triggered and internally generated inhibition identify a neural mechanism of will. *Journal of Cognitive Neuroscience*, *27*, 1948–1956.

Passingham, R. E., Rowe, J. B., & Sakai, K. (2012). Has brain imaging discovered anything new about how the brain works? *NeuroImage, 66,* 142–150.

Pauli, W. M., O'Reilly, R. C., Yarkoni, T., & Wager, T. D. (2016). Regional specialization within the human striatum for diverse psychological functions. *Proceedings of the National Academy of Sciences of the United States of America, 113,* 1907–1912.

Pecina, M., Bohnert, A. S., Sikora, M., Avery, E. T., Langenecker, S. A., Mickey, B. J., et al. (2015). Placebo-activated neural systems are linked to antidepressant responses. *JAMA Psychiatry, 72,* 1087–1094.

Pellis, S. M., O'Brien, D. P., Pellis, V. C., Teitelbaum, P., Wolgin, D. L., & Kennedy, S. (1988). Escalation of feline predation along a gradient from avoidance through "play" to killing. *Behavioral Neuroscience, 102,* 760–777.

Penn, D. C., Holyoak, K. J., & Povenelli, D. J. (2008). Darwin's mistake: Explaining the discontinuity between human and nonhuman animals. *Behavioral and Brain Sciences, 31,* 109–130.

Penn, J. K. M., Zito, M. F., & Kravitz, E. A. (2010). A single social defeat reduces aggression in a highly aggressive strain of *Drosophila. Proceedings of the National Academy of Sciences of the United States of America, 107,* 12862–12866.

Perera, T., George, M. S., Grammer, G., Janicak, P. G., Pascual-Leone, A., & Wirecki, T. S. (2016). The clinical TMS society consensus review and treatment recommendations for TMS therapy for major depressive disorder. *Brain Stimulation,* Mar 16. pii:S1935–861X (16)30038–9.

Perri, R. L., Berchicci, M., Lucci, G., Cimmino, R. L., Bello, A., & Di Russo, F. (2014). Getting ready for an emotion. *Frontiers in Behavioral Neuroscience, 8,* 197–205.

Peters, L., Polspoel, B., Op de Beeck, H., & De Smedt, B. (2016). Brain activity during arithmetic in symbolic and non-symbolic formats in 9–12 year old children. *Neuropsychologia, 86,* 19–28.

Petersen, S., Schroijen, M., Molders, C., Zenker, S., & Van den Bergh, O. (2014). Categorical interoception: Perceptual organization of sensations from inside. *Psychological Science*, *25*, 1059–1066.

Pfaff, D. W. (2015). *The altruistic brain*. New York: Oxford University Press.

Phillips, D., Gormley, W., & Anderson, S. (2016). Tulsa's CAP Head Start program and middle-school academic outcomes and processes. *Developmental Psychology*, *52*, 1247–1261.

Piaget, J. (1950). *Psychology of intelligence*. London: Routledge and Kegan Paul.

Piantadosi, S. T., & Kidd, C. (2016). Extraordinary intelligence and the care of infants. *Proceedings of the National Academy of Sciences of the United States of America*, *113*, 6874–6879.

Piantadosi, S. T., Kidd, C., & Aslin, R. (2014). Rich analysis and rational models. *Developmental Science*, *17*, 321–337.

Pichel, B. (2016). From facial expressions to bodily gestures. *History of the Human Sciences*, *29*, 27–48.

Pitcher, B. J., Mesoudi, A., & McElligott, A. G. (2013). Sex-biased sound symbolism in English-language first names. *PLoS One*, *8*, e64825.

Poldrack, R. A., & Yarkoni, T. (2016). From brain to cognitive ontologies. *Annual Review of Psychology*, *67*, 587–612.

Pollen, D. A. (2011). On the emergence of primary visual perception. *Cerebral Cortex*, *21*, 1941–1953.

Popper, K. R., & Eccles, J. C. (1977). *The self and its brain*. New York: Springer-Verlag.

Pornpattananangkul, N., Hariri, A. R., Harada, T., Mano, Y., Komeda, H., Parrish, T. B., Sadato, N., Iidaka, T., & Chiao, J. Y. (2016). Cultural influences on neural basis of inhibitory control. *NeuroImage*, *139*, 114–126.

Porter, K. B. (2016). *The road to success* (Unpublished doctoral dissertation). Harvard University, Cambridge, MA.

Porto, F. H. G., Tusch, E. S., Fox, A. M., Alperin, B. R., Holcomb, P. H., & Daffner, K. R. (2016). One of the most well-established age-related changes in neural activity disappears after controlling for visual acuity. *NeuroImage*, *130*, 115–122.

Potts, J. T., & Mitchell, J. H. (1998). Rapid resetting of carotid baroceptor reflex by afferent input from skeletal muscle receptors. *American Journal of Physiology*, *275*, H2000–H2008.

Prins, S. J., Bates, L. M., Keyes, K. M., & Muntaner, C. (2015). Anxious? Depressed? You might be suffering from capitalism. *Sociology of Health & Illness*, *37*, 1352–1372.

Putnam, H. (2012). *Philosophy in an age of science*. Cambridge, MA: Harvard University Press.

Quellet, M., Santiago, J., Funes, M. J., & Lupianez, J. (2010). Thinking about the future moves attention to the right. *Journal of Experimental Psychology: Human Perception and Performance*, *36*, 17–24.

Rajalingham, R., Stacey, R. G., Tsoulfas, G., & Musallam, S. (2014). Modulation of neural activity by reward in medial intraparietal cortex is sensitive to temporal sequence of reward. *Journal of Neurophysiology*, *112*, 1775–1789.

Rajimehr, R., Devaney, K. J., Bilenko, N. Y., Young, J. C., & Tootell, R. B. H. (2011). The "parahippocampal place area" responds preferentially to high spatial frequencies in humans and monkeys. *PLoS Biology*, *9*, e1000608.

Rajkumar, A. P., Brinda, E. M., Duba, A. S., Thangadurai, P., & Jacob, K. S. (2013). National suicide rates and mental health system indicators: An ecological study of 191 countries. *International Journal of Law and Psychiatry*, *36*, 339–342.

Ramenzoni, V. C., & Liszowski, U. (2016). The social reach. *Psychological Science*, *27*, 1278–1285.

Ranganath, C., & Rainer, G. (2003). Neural mechanisms for detecting and remembering novel events. *Nature Reviews. Neuroscience*, *4*, 193–202.

Raphael, S., & Morgan, M. J. (2016). The computation of relative numerosity, size and density. *Vision Research, 124*, 15–23.

Rath, J., Wurnig, M., Fischmeister, F., Klinger, N., Hollinger, I., Geibler, A., et al. (2016). Between- and within-site variability of fMRI localizations. *Human Brain Mapping, 37*, 2151–2160.

Reggev, N., Bein, O., & Maril, A. (2016). Distinct neural suppression and encoding effects for conceptual novelty and familiarity. *Journal of Cognitive Neuroscience, 28*, 1455–1470.

Reilly, J., Westbury, C., Kean, J., & Peelle, J. E. (2012). Arbitrary symbolism in natural language revisited. *PLoS One, 7*, e42286.

Rekkas, P. V., & Constable, R. T. (2006). Hemodynamic retrieval intensity in hippocampus is decreased by pre-exposure to autobiographical test items. *Brain Research Bulletin, 70*, 467–473.

Rentfrow, P. J., Jakela, M., & Lamb, M. E. (2015). Regional personality differences in Great Britain. *PLoS One, 10*, e122245.

Rescorla, R. A., & Wagner, A. R. (1972). A theory of Pavlovian conditioning. In A. H. Black & W. F. Prokasy (Eds.), *Classical conditioning II: Current research and theory* (pp. 64–99). New York: Appleton-Century-Crofts.

Reuter, M., Tisdall, M. D., Qureshi, A., Buckner, R. L., van der Kouwe, A. J., & Fischi, B. (2015). Head motion during MRI acquisition reduces gray matter volume and thickness estimates. *NeuroImage, 107*, 107–115.

Rhudy, J. L., Williams, A. E., McCabe, K. M., Rambo, P. L., & Russell, J. L. (2006). Emotional modulation of spinal nociception and pain. *Pain, 126*, 221–233.

Richmond, J. L., Zhao, J. L., & Burns, M. A. (2015). What goes where? Eye tracking reveals spatial relational memory during infancy. *Journal of Experimental Child Psychology, 130*, 79–91.

Rigoli, F., Chew, B., Dayan, P., & Dolan, R. J. (2016). The dopaminergic midbrain mediates an effect of average reward on Pavlovian vigor. *Journal of Cognitive Neuroscience, 28*, 1303–1317.

Rilling, J. K., Demarco, A. C., Hackett, P. D., Chen, X., Gautam, P., Stair, S., et al. (2014). Sex differences in the neural and behavioral response to intranasal oxytocin and vasopressin during human social interaction. *Psychoendocrinology, 39,* 10–16.

Rissman, J., Chow, T. E., Reggente, N., & Wagner, A. D. (2016). Decoding fMRI signatures of real-world autobiographical memory retrieval. *Journal of Cognitive Neuroscience, 28,* 604–620.

Rizzolatti, G., & Craighero, L. (2004). The mirror-neuron system. *Annual Review of Neuroscience, 27,* 169–192.

Rizzolatti, G., & Sinigaglia, C. (2016). The mirror mechanism. *Nature Reviews. Neuroscience, 17,* 757–765.

Roberts, A. L., Rosario, M., Slopen, N., Calzo, J. P., & Austin, S. B. (2013). Childhood gender nonconformity, bullying, victimization, and depressive symptoms across adolescence and early adulthood. *Journal of the American Academy of Child and Adolescent Psychiatry, 52,* 143–152.

Robertson, D. R. (1972). Social control of sex reversal in a coral-reef fish. *Science, 177,* 1007–1009.

Rodger, H., Vizioli, L., Ouyang, X., & Caldera, R. (2015). Mapping the development of facial expression recognition. *Developmental Science, 18,* 926–939.

Rommers, J., Dijkstra, T., & Bastiaansen, M. (2013). Context-dependent semantic processing in the human brain. *Journal of Cognitive Neuroscience, 25,* 762–776.

Roy, B. C., Frank, M. C., DeCamp, P., Miller, M., & Roy, D. (2015). Predicting the birth of a spoken word. *Proceedings of the National Academy of Sciences of the United States of America, 112,* 12663–12668.

Rubin, D. C., & Kozin, M. (1984). Vivid memories. *Cognition, 16,* 81–95.

Ruff, D. A., & Cohen, M. R. (2016). Stimulus dependence of correlated variability across cortical areas. *Journal of Neuroscience, 36,* 7546–7556.

Rupia, E. J., Binning, S. A., Roche, D. G., & Lu, W. (2016). Fight-flight or freeze-hide? Personality and metabolic phenotype mediate physiological defence responses in flatfish. *Journal of Animal Ecology*, *85*, 927–937. doi:10.1111/1365-2656.12524.

Saarimaki, H., Gotsopoulos, A., Jaaskelainen, I. P., Lampinen, J., Vuilleumier, P., Hari, R., et al. (2016). Discrete neural signatures of basic emotions. *Cerebral Cortex*, *26*, 2563–2573.

Sabuncu, M. R., Ge, T., Holmes, A. J., Smoller, J. W., Buckner, R. L., & Fischl, B. (2016). Morphometricity as a measure of the neuroanatomical signature of a trait. *Proceedings of the National Academy of Sciences of the United States of America*, *113*, E5749–E5756.

Salamone, J. D., Correa, M., Farrar, A., & Mingote, S. M. (2007). Effort-related functions of nucleus accumbens dopamine and associated forebrain circuits. *Psychopharmacology*, *191*, 461–482.

Salomon, R., Ronchi, R., Donz, J., Bello-Ruiz, J., Herbelin, B., Martet, R., et al. (2016). The insula mediates access to awareness of the visual stimuli presented synchronously to the heartbeat. *Journal of Neuroscience*, *36*, 5115–5127.

Salz, D. M., Tiganj, Z., Khasnabish, S., Kohley, A., Sheehan, D., Howard, M. W., et al. (2016). Time cells in hippocampal area CA3. *Journal of Neuroscience*, *36*, 7476–7484.

Sariaslan, A., Larsson, H., & Fazel, S. (2016). Genetic and environmental determinants of violence risk in psychotic disorders. *Molecular Psychiatry*, *21*, 1251–1256.

Sarinopoulos, I., Grupe, D. W., Mackiewicz, K. L., Herrington, J. D., Lor, M., Steege, E. E., & Nitschke, J. (2010). Uncertainty during anticipation modulates neural responses to aversion in human insula and amygdala. *Cerebral Cortex*, *20*, 929–940.

Savage, R. A., Becker, S., & Lipp, O. V. (2016). Visual search for emotional expressions: Effect of stimulus set on anger and happiness superiority. *Cognition and Emotion*, *30*, 713–730.

Scarf, D., Boy, K., Reinert, A. U., Devine, J., Gunturkun, O., & Colombo, M. (2016). Orthographic processing in pigeons (*Columba* livia). *Proceedings of the National Academy of Sciences of the United States of America, 113*, 11272–11276.

Schacter, D. L. (1999). The seven sins of memory. *American Psychologist, 54*, 182–203.

Schacter, S., & Singer, J. E. (1962). Cognitive, social, and physiological determinants of emotional states. *Psychological Review, 69*, 379–399.

Schafer, A., Schienle, A., & Vaitl, D. (2005). Stimulus type and design influence hemodynamic response towards visual disgust and fear elicitors. *International Journal of Psychophysiology, 57*, 53–59.

Scheel, D., Godfrey-Smith, P., & Lawrence, M. (2016). Signal use by octopuses in agonistic interactions. *Current Biology, 26*, 377–382.

Scheele, D., Striepens, N., Kendrick, K. M., Schwering, C., Noelle, J., Wille, A., et al. (2014). Opposing effects of oxytocin on moral judgment in males and females. *Human Brain Mapping, 35*, 6067–6076. doi:10.1002/hbm.22605.

Scherer, K. R. (1997). Profiles of emotion-antecedent appraisal. *Cognition and Emotion, 11*, 113–150.

Schienle, A., Ubels, S., Schongasner, F., Ille, R., & Scharmuller, W. (2013). Disgust regulation via placebo. *Social Cognitive and Affective Neuroscience, 9*, 985–990.

Schiff, M., Duyme, M., Dumaret, A., Stewart, J., Tomkiewicz, S., & Feingold, J. (1978). Intellectual status of working-class children adopted early into upper-middle class families. *Science, 200*, 1503–1504.

Schindler, S., & Kissler, J. (2016). People matter. *NeuroImage, 134*, 160–169.

Schindler, S., Wegrzyn, M., Steppacher, I., & Kissler, J. (2015). Perceived communicative context and emotional content amplify visual word processing in the fusiform gyrus. *Journal of Neuroscience, 35*, 6010–6019.

Schmandt-Besserat, D. (1996). *How writing came about.* Austin, TX: University of Texas Press.

Schnohr, C. W., Gobina, I., Santos, T., Mazur, J., Alikasifuglu, M., Valimaa, R. Torsheim, T. (2016). Semantic bias in cross-national comparative analysis. *Health Quality Life Outcomes*, *14*(1), 70.

Schultz, W. (2015). Neural reward and decision signals. *Physiological Reviews*, *95*, 853–951.

Schurer, R. K. (2016). *Seeing motion*. Berlin: De Gruyter.

Schuster, S., Hawelka, S., Hutzler, F., Kronbichler, M., & Richlan, F. (2016). Words in context. *Cerebral Cortex*, *26*, 3889–3904.

Schwartz, C. E., Kunwar, P. S., Greve, D. N., Kagan, J., Snidman, N. C., & Bloch, R. B. (2012). A phenotype of early infancy predicts reactivity of the amygdala in male adults. *Molecular Psychiatry*, *17*, 1042–1050.

Schwarz, K. A., Pfister, R., & Buchel, C. (2016). Rethinking explicit expectations. *Trends in Cognitive Sciences*, *20*, 469–481.

Schwerdtfeger, A. R. (2004). Predicting autonomic reactivity to public speaking: Don't get fixed on self-report. *International Journal of Psychophysiology*, *52*, 217–224.

Scott, K. M., Smith, D. A. R., & Ellis, P. M. (2012). A population study of childhood maltreatment and asthma diagnosis. *Psychosomatic Medicine*, *74*, 817–823.

Searle, J. (2003). Putting consciousness back in the brain. In M. Bennett, D. Dennett, P. Hacker, & J. Searle (Eds.), *Neuroscience and philosophy* (pp. 97–124). New York: Columbia University Press.

Segre, G., & Hoerlin, B. (2016). *The pope of physics*. New York: Henry Holt.

Sera-Shriar, E. (2015). Anthropometric portraiture and Victorian anthropology. *History of Science*, *53*, 155–179.

Setoh, P., Scott, R. M., & Baillargeon, R. (2016). Two-and-a-half-year-olds succeed at a traditional false-belief task with reduced processing demands. *Proceedings of the National Academy of Sciences of the United States of America*, *113*, 13360–13365.

Shackman, A. J., & Fox, A. S. (2016). Contributions of the central extended amygdala to fear and anxiety. *Journal of Neuroscience, 36,* 8050–8063.

Shafir, S., & Barron, A. B. (2010). Optic flow informs distance but not profitability. *Proceedings. Biological Sciences, 277,* 1241–1245.

Sharan, P., Sundar, A. S., Thennarasu, K., & Reddy, Y. C. (2015). Is late-onset OCD a distinct phenotype? *CNS Spectrums, 20,* 508–514.

Sharif, M. A., & Oppenheimer, D. M. (2016). The effect of relative encoding on memory-based judgments. *Psychological Science, 27,* 1136–1145.

Sharpe, D., & Whelton, W. J. (2016). Frightened by an old scarecrow: The remarkable resilience of demand characteristics. *Review of General Psychology, 20,* 349–368.

Sheehan, H. R., & Franklin, D. W. (2016). Motor planning, not execution, separates motor memories. *Neuron, 92,* 773–779.

Shelton, M. M., Schminkey, D. L., & Groer, M. W. (2015). Relationships among prenatal depression, plasma cortisol, and inflammatory cytokines. *Biological Research for Nursing, 17,* 295–302.

Sherman, M. T., Kanai, R., Seth, A. K., & VanRullen, R. (2016). Rhythmic influences of top-down perceptual priors in the phase of prestimulus occipital alpha oscillations. *Journal of Cognitive Neuroscience, 28,* 1318–1330.

Shibata, K., Sasaki, Y., Kawato, M., & Watanabe, T. (2016). Neuro-imaging evidence for 2 types of plasticity in association with visual perceptual learning. *Cerebral Cortex, 26,* 3681–3689.

Shields, P. J., & Rovee-Collier, C. (1992). Long-term memory for context-specific category information at six months. *Child Development, 63,* 245–259.

Shine, J. M., Koyejo, O., & Poldrack, R. A. (2016). Temporal metastates are associated with differential patterns of time-resolved connectivity, network topology, and attention. *Proceedings of the National Academy of Sciences of the United States of America, 113*, 9888–9891.

Shutts, K., Brey, E. L., Dornbusch, L. A., Slywotzky, N., & Olson, K. R. (2016). Children use wealth cues to evaluate others. *PLoS One, 11*, e0149360.

Sidhu, D, M., & Pexman, P. M. (2015). What's in a name? Sound symbolism and gender in first names. *PLoS One, 10*(5), e0126809.

Siegler, R. S. (2016). Magnitude knowledge: The common core of numerical development. *Developmental Science, 19*, 341–360.

Sigelman, C. K., & Waitzman, K. A. (1991). The development of a distributive justice orientation. *Child Development, 62*, 1367–1378.

Silva, K., Chein, J., & Steinberg, L. (2016). Adolescents in peer groups make more prudent decisions when a slightly older adult is present. *Psychological Science, 27*, 322–330.

Silvers, J. A., Insel, C., Powers, A., Franz, P., Helion, C., Martin, R., Weber, J., Mischel, W., Casey, B. J., & Ochsner, K. N. (2016). The transition from childhood to adolescence is marked by a general decrease in amygdala reactivity and an affect-specific ventral-to-dorsal shift in medial prefrontal recruitment. *Developmental Cognitive Neuroscience*, pii:S1878–9293(16)30072-X doi:10.1016/j.dcn. 2016.06.005.

Sinatra, R., Wang, D., Deville, P., Song, C., & Barabasi, A. L. (2016). Quantifying the evolution of individual scientific impact. *Science, 354*, 596.

Singer, T., Seymour, B., O'Doherty, J., Kaube, H., Dolan, R. J., & Frith, C. D. (2004). Empathy for pain involves the affective but not sensory components of pain. *Science, 303*, 1157–1162.

Singh, L., & Fu, C. S. L. (2016). A new view of language development: The acquisition of lexical tone. *Child Development, 87*, 834–854.

Sinke, C., Forkmann, K., Schmidt, K., Wiech, K., & Bingel, U. (2016). Expectations impact short-term memory through changes in connectivity between attention- and task-related brain regions. *Cortex, 78*, 1–14.

Smith, R. (1992). *Inhibition*. Berkeley, CA: University of California Press.

Smith, A. K., Rhee, S. H., Corley, R. P., Friedman, N. P., Hewitt, J. K., & Robinson, J. A. L. (2013). The magnitude of genetic and environmental influences on parental and observational measures of behavioral inhibition and shyness in toddlerhood. *Behavior Genetics, 42*, 764–777.

Smith, K. S., & Graybiel, A. M. (2016). Habit formation coincides with shifts in reinforcement representations in the sensorimotor striatum. *Journal of Neurophysiology, 115*, 1487–1498.

Solomon, R. L., & Wynne, L. C. (1953). Traumatic avoidance learning. *Psychological Monographs, 67*, 1–19.

Song, L., Pruden, S. M., Golinkoff, R. M., & Hirsh-Pasek, K. (2016). Prelinguistic foundations of verb learning. *Journal of Experimental Child Psychology*. doi:10.1016/j.jecp.2016.01.004.

Sood, M. R., & Sereno, M. I. (2016). Areas activated during naturalistic reading comprehension L overlap topological visual, auditory, and somatomotor maps. *Human Brain Mapping, 37*, 2784–2810.

Sorenson, D. A., McManis, M., & Kagan, J. (2002). Emotion, cognition, and startle reflex modulation (Unpublished manuscript).

Soussignan, R., & Schall, B. (1996). Children's facial responsiveness to odors. *Developmental Psychology, 32*, 367–379.

Spaapen, D. L., Waters, F., Brummer, L., Stopa, L., & Bucks, R. S. (2014). The emotion regulation questionnaire: Validation of the ERQ-9 in two community samples. *Psychological Assessment, 26*, 46–54.

Spetch, M. L., & Parent, M. B. (2006). Age and sex differences in children's spatial search strategies. *Psychonomic Bulletin & Review, 13*, 807–812.

Spiers, H., Hannon, E., Schalkwyk, L. C., Smith, R., Wong, C. C., O'Donovan, M. C., et al. (2015). Methylomic trajectories across human fetal brain development. *Genome Research, 25*, 338–352.

Spironelli, C., Busenello, J., & Angrilli, A. (2016). Supine posture inhibits cortical activity. *Neuropsychologia, 89*, 125–131.

Srihasam, K., Vincent, J. L., & Livingstone, M. S. (2014). Novel domain formation reveals proto-architecture in inferotemporal cortex. *Nature Neuroscience, 17,* 1776–1783.

Srinivasan, R., Golomb, J. D., & Martinez, A. M. (2016). A neural basis of facial action recognition in humans. *Journal of Neuroscience, 36,* 4434–4442.

Steenrod, S. C., Phillips, M. H., & Goldberg, M. E. (2013). The lateral intraparietal area codes the location of saccade targets and not the dimension of the saccades that will be made to acquire them. *Journal of Neurophysiology, 109,* 2596–2605.

Stein, M. B., Chen, C. Y., Ursano, R. J., Cai, T., Gelertner, J., Heeringa, S. G., et al. (2016). Genome-wide association studies of Posttraumatic Stress Disorder in 2 cohorts of US Army soldiers. *JAMA Psychiatry, 73,* 695–704.

Stephenson, A. R., Edler, M. K., Erwin, J. M., Jacobs, B., Hopkins, W. D., Hof, P. R., et al. (2017). Cholinergic innervation of the basal ganglia in humans and other anthropoid prinates. *Journal of Comparative Neurology, 525,* 319–332.

Stewart, A. J., Parsons, T. L., & Plotkin, J. B. (2016). Evolutionary consequences of behavioral diversity. *Proceedings of the National Academy of Sciences of the United States of America, 113,* E7003–E7009.

Stimpson, C. D., Tetreault, N. A., Allman, J. M., Jacobs, B., Butti, C., Hof, P. R., & Sherwood, C. C. (2011). Biochemical specificity of von Economo neurons in hominids. *American Journal of Human Biology, 23,* 22–28.

Stotz, S. J., Elbert, T., Muller, V., & Schauer, M. (2015). The relationship between trauma, shame, and guilt. *European Journal of Psychotraumatology, 6.* doi:3402/ejpt.v6. 25867.

Strange, B. A., & Dolan, R. J. (2001). Adaptive anterior hippocampal responses to oddball stimuli. *Hippocampus, 11,* 690–698.

Strawson, G. (2013). Real naturalism. *London Review of Books,* Sep 26, 28–30.

Striano, T., & Bushnell, E. W. (2005). Haptic perception of material properties by 3-month-old infants. *Infant Behavior and Development, 28,* 266–289.

Subramanian, H. H., Arun, M., Silburn, P., & Holstege, G. (2015). The motor organization of positive and negative emotional vocalization in the cat midbrain periaqueductal gray. *Journal of Comparative Neurology, 524*(8), 1540–1557. doi:1002.cne.23869.

Suchak, M., Eppley, T. M., Campbell, M. W., Feldman, R. A., Quarles, L. F., & de Waal, F. B. (2016). How chimpanzees cooperate in a competitive world. *Proceedings of the National Academy of Sciences of the United States of America, 113,* 10215–10220.

Sulovari, A., Kranzler, H. R., Farrer, L. A., Gelernter, J., & Li, D. (2015). Further analyses support the association between light eye color and alcohol dependence. *American Journal of Medical Genetics. Part B, Neuropsychiatric Genetics, 168,* 757–760.

Sussman, E. S., Chen, S., Sussman-Fort, J., & Dinces, E. (2014). The five myths of MMN. *Brain Topography, 27,* 553–564.

Swaminathan, S., MacSweeney, M., Boyles, R., Waters, D., Watkins, K. E., & Mottonen, R. (2013). Motor excitability during visual perception of known and unknown spoken language. *Brain and Language, 126,* 1–7.

Swartz, J. R., Hariri, A. R., & Williamson, P. E. (20160. An epigenetic mechanisms links socioeconomic status to changes in depression-related brain function in high-risk adolescents. *Molecular Psychiatry.* doi:10.1038/mp.2016.82.

Swettenham, J. B., Muthukumaraswamy, S. D., & Singh, K. D. (2013). BOLD responses in human primary visual cortex are insensitive to substantial changes in neural activity. *Frontiers in Human Neuroscience, 7,* 76. doi:10.3389/fnhumns.

Swift, H. J., Vauclair, C. M., Abrams, D., Bratt, C., Marques, S., & Lima, M. L. (2014). Revisiting the paradox of well-being. *Journals of Gerontology. Series B, Psychological Sciences and Social Sciences, 69,* 920–932.

Taggart, P., Sutton, P. M., Groves, D., Holdright, D. R., Bradbury, D., Brill, D., & Critchley, H. (2007). A cortical potential reflecting cardiac function. *Proceedings of the National Academy of Sciences of the United States of America, 104*, 6818–6820.

Tai, S. K., & Leung, L. S. (2012). Vestibular stimulation enhances hippocampal long-term potentiation via activation of cholinergic septohippocampal cells. *Behavioural Brain Research, 232*, 174–182.

Takahashi, Y. K., Langdon, A. J., Niv, Y., & Schoenbaum, G. (2016). Temporal specificity of reward prediction error signaled by putative dopamine neurons in rat VTA depends on ventral striatum. *Neuron, 91*, 182–193.

Takeuchi, T., Duszkiewicz, A. J., Sonneborn, A., Spooner, D. A., Yamasaki, Y., Watanabe, M., et al. (2016). Locus coereleus and dopaminergic consolidation of everyday memory. *Nature, 537*, 357–362.

Takuyama, N., & Furuichi, T. (2016). Do females help each other? Patterns of female coalition formation in wild bonobos in Wamba. *Animal Behaviour, 119*, 27–35.

Taleb, N. N. (2007). *The black swan.* New York: Random House.

Tamir, D. I., Thornton, M. A., Contreras, J. M., & Mitchell, J. P. (2016). Neural evidence that three dimensions organize mental state representations: Rationality, social impact, and valence. *Proceedings of the National Academy of Sciences of the United States of America, 113*, 194–199.

Tamir, M., Schwartz, S. H., Cieciuch, J., Riedeger, M., Torres, C., Scollon, C., et al. (2016). Desired emotions across cultures: A value-based account. *Journal of Personality and Social Psychology, 111*, 67–82.

Taquet, M., Quoidbach, J., de Montjoye, Y. A., Desseilles, M., & Gross, J. J. (2016). Hedonism and the choice of everyda activties. *Proceedings of the National Academy of Sciences of the United States of America, 113*, 9769–9773.

Teigen, K. H. (1985). Preference for news as a function of familiarity. *Scandinavian Journal of Psychology, 26*, 348–356.

Thibault, R. T., Lifshitz, M., & Raz, A. (2016). Body position alters human resting-state: Insights from multi-postural magnetoencephalography. *Brain Imaging and Behavior, 10,* 772–780.

Thoresen, S., Jensen, T. K., Wentzel-Larsen, T., & Dyb, G. (2016). Parents of terror victims. *Journal of Anxiety Disorders, 38,* 47–54.

Thorndike, E. L. (1898). Animal intelligence. *Psychological Monographs, 2,* i-119.

Tian, J., Huang, R., Cohen, J. Y., Osakada, F., Kobak, D., Machens, C. K., et al. (2016). Distributed and mixed information in monosynaptic inputs to dopamine neurons. *Neuron, 91,* 1374–1389.

Timm, J., Schonwieser, M., Schroger, E., & San Miguel, I. (2016). Sensory suppression of brain response to self-generated sounds is observed with and without the perception of agency. *Cortex,* Apr 2. pii:S00100452.

Tolman, E. C. (1932). *Purposive behavior in animals and men.* New York: Appleton-Century-Crofts.

Tolman, E. C. (1938). The determiners of behavior at a choice point. *Psychological Review, 45,* 1–41.

Tomasello, M. (2016). *A natural history of human morality.* Cambridge, MA: Harvard University Press.

Tomasello, M., Call, J., & Gluckman, A. (1997). Comprehension of novel communicative signs by apes and human children. *Child Development, 68,* 1067–1080.

Tomasi, D., & Volkow, N. D. (2012). Laterality patterns of brain functional connectivity: Gender effects. *Cerebral Cortex, 22,* 1455–1462.

Tomkins, S. S. (1962). *The positive affects.* New York: Springer.

Tomkins, S. S. (1963). *The negative affects.* New York: Springer.

Torralbo, A., Walther, D. B., Chai, B., Caddigan, E., Fei-Fei, L., & Beck, D. M. (2013). Good exemplars of natural scene categories elicit clearer patterns than bad exemplars but not greater BOLD activity. *PLoS One, 8,* e58594.

Torrents-Rodas, D., Fullana, M. A., Bunillo, A., Caseras, X., Andian, O., & Torruba, R. (2013). No effect of trait anxiety on differential fear conditioning or fear generalization. *Biological Psychology, 92*, 185–190.

Tourangeau, R. (2007). Sensitive questions in surveys. *Psychological Bulletin, 133*, 859–883.

Tovote, P., Esposito, M. S., Botta, R., Chaudun, E., Fadok, J. P., Marokovic, M., et al. (2016). Midbrain circuits for defensive behavior. *Nature, 534*, 206–212.

Trappler, B., Cohen, C. I., & Tulloo, R. (2007). Impact of early lifetime trauma in later life. *American Journal of Geriatric Psychiatry, 15*, 79–83.

Trinh, N. H., Nadler, D. L., Shie, V., Fregni, F., Gilman, S. E., Ryan, C. M., & Schneider, J. C. (2014). Psychological sequelae of the station nightclub fire. *PLoS One, 9*, e115013.

Trisko, R. K., Sandel, A. A., & Smuts, B. (2016). Affiliation, dominance and friendship among companion dogs. *Behaviour*. doi:10.1163/1568539.

Trueblood, J. S., Brown, S. D., Heathcote, A., & Busemeyer, J. R. (2013). Not just for consumers: Context effects are fundamental to decision making. *Psychological Science, 24*, 901–908.

Tudusciuc, O., & Nieder, A. (2009). Contributions of primate prefrontal and posterior parietal cortices to length and numerosity representations. *Journal of Neurophysiology, 101*, 2984–2994.

Tukey, J. W. (1969). Analyzing data: Sanctification or detective work? *American Psychologist, 24*, 83–91.

Turgeon, S. M. (2008). Sex differences in children's face drawings and their relationship to 2D:4D ratio. *Personality and Individual Differences, 45*, 527–532.

Turkheimer, E., Haley, A., Waldron, M., D'Onofrio, B., & Gottesman, I. I. (2003). Socioeconomic status modifies heritability of IQ in young children. *Psychological Science, 14*, 623–628.

Twenge, J. M., Campbell, W. K., & Carter, N. T. (2014). Declines in trust in others and confidence in institutions among American adults and late adolescents. *Psychological Science*, *25*, 1914–1923.

Tylen, K., Philipsen, J. S., Roepstorff, A., & Fusaroli, R. (2016). Trails of meaning construction. *NeuroImage*, *134*, 105–112.

Ulber, J., Hamann, K., & Tomasello, M. (2016). Young children, but not chimpanzees, are averse to disadvantageous and advantageous inequities. *Journal of Experimental Child Psychology*, *155*, 48–66.

Uttal, W. R. (2011). *Mind and brain*. Cambridge, MA: MIT Press.

Vachon-Presseau, E., Roy, M., Martel, M. O., Albouy, G., Chen, J., Budell, L., et al. (2012). Neural processing of sensory and emotional-communicative information associated with the perception of vicarious pain. *NeuroImage*, *63*, 54–62.

Van Bavel, J. J., Mende-Siedlecki, P., Brady, W. J., & Reinero, D. A. (2016). Contextual sensitivity in scientific reproducibility. *Proceedings of the National Academy of Sciences of the United States of America*, *113*, 6454–6459.

Van Dam, W. O., van Dongen, E. V., Bekkering, H., & Rueschemeyer, S. A. (2012). Context-dependent changes in functional connectivity of auditory cortices during the perception of object words. *Journal of Cognitive Neuroscience*, *24*, 2108–2119.

Vandekar, S. N., Shinohara, R. T., Raznahan, A., Hopson, R. D., Roalf, D. R., Ruparel, K., et al. (2016). Subject-level measurement of local cortical coupling. *NeuroImage*, *133*, 88–97.

Vandenbroucke, A. R. E., Fahrenfort, J. J., Meuwese, D. I., Scholte, H. S., & Lamme, V. A. F. (2016). Prior knowledge about objects determines neural color representation in human visual cortex. *Cerebral Cortex*, *26*, 1401–1408.

Van Leeuwen, E. J., Mulenga, I. C., Bodamer, M. D., & Cronin, K. A. (2016). Chimpanzees' responses to the dead body of a 9-year-old group member. *American Journal of Primatology*, *78*, 914–922.

Van Maanen, L., Forstmann, B. U., Keuken, M. C., Wagenmakers, E. J., & Heathcote, A. (2016). The impact of MRI scanner environment on perceptual decision making. *Behavior Research Methods, 48*, 184–200.

Van Renswoude, D. R., Johnson, S. P., Raijmakers, M. E., & Visser, I. (2016). Do infants have the horizontal bias? *Infant Behavior and Development, 44*, 38–48.

Van Strien, J. W., Christiaans, G., Franken, I. H., & Huijding, J. (2016). Curvilinear shapes and the snake detection hypothesis: An ERP study. *Psychophysiology, 53*, 252–257.

Vaughn, B. E., Joffe, L. S., Bradley, C. F., Seifer, R., & Barglow, P. (1987). Maternal characteristics measured prenatally are predictive of ratings of temperamental "difficulty" on the Carey Infant Temperament Questionnaire. *Developmental Psychology, 23*, 152–161.

Vaughn-Coaxum, R. A., Mair, P., & Weisz, J. R. (2016). Racial/ethnic differences in youth depression indicators. *Clinical Psychological Science, 4*, 239–253.

Veale, D., Eshkevari, E., Read, J., Miles, S., Troglia, A., Phillips, R., et al. (2014). Beliefs about penis size. *Journal of Sexual Medicine, 11*, 84–92.

Venkatesh, S. A. (2013). *Floating city*. New York: Penguin Press.

Verbaarschot, C., Haselager, P., & Farquhar, J. (2016). Detecting traces of consciousness in the process of intending to act. *Experimental Brain Research, 234*, 1945–1956.

Vernon, R. J. W., Gouws, A. D., Lawrence, S. J. D., Wade, A. R., & Morland, A. B. (2016). Multivariate patterns in the human object-processing pathway reveal a shift from retinotopic to shape curvature representations in lateral occipital areas, LO-1 and LO-2. *Journal of Neuroscience, 36*, 5763–5774.

Veroude, K., Zhang-James, Y., Fernandez-Castillo, N., Bakker, M. J., & Cormand, B. (2016). Genetics of aggressive behavior: An overview. *American Journal of Medical Genetics. Part B, Neuropsychiatric Genetics, 171*, 3–43.

Vertes, R. P., Linley, S. B., & Hoover, W. B. (2015). Limbic circuitry of the midbrain thalamus. *Neuroscience and Biobehavioral Reviews, 54*, 89–107.

Vervaecke, H., de Vries, H., & van Elsacker, L. (1999). An experimental evaluation of the consistency of competitive ability and agnostic dominance in different social contexts in captive bonobos. *Behavior Genetics, 136*, 423–442.

Vied, C., Ray, S., Badger, C. D., Bundy, J. L., Arbeitman, M. N., & Nowakowski, R. S. (2016). Transcriptomic analysis of the hippocampus from six inbred strains of mice suggest a basis for sex-specific susceptibility and severity of neurological disorders. *Journal of Comparative Neurology, 524*, 2696–2710.

Vinken, K., Van den Bergh, G., Vermaercke, B., & Op de Beeck, H. (2016). Neural representations of natural and scrambled movies progressively change from rat striate to temporal cortex. *Cerebral Cortex, 26*, 3310–3322.

Vogel, A., & La Salle, J. A. (2016). The landscape of DNA methylation amid a perfect storm of autism aetiologies. *Nature Reviews. Neuroscience, 17*, 411–423.

Volk, D. W., Sampson, A. R., Zhang, Y., Edelson, J. R., & Lewis, D. A. (2016). Cortical GABA markers identify a molecular subtype of psychotic and bipolar disorders. *Psychological Medicine, 46*, 2501–2512.

Volter, C. J., Sentis, I., & Call, J. (2016). Great apes and children infer causal relations from patterns of variation and covariation. *Cognition, 155*, 30–43.

Vrticka, P., Lordier, L., Bediou, B., & Sander, D. (2014). Human amygdala responses to dynamic facial expressions of positive and negative surprise. *Emotion, 14*, 161–169.

Wagemans, J., Elder, J. H., Kubovy, M., Palmer, S. E., Peterson, M. A., Singh, M., & von der Heydt (2012). A century of Gestalt psychology in visual perception: I. Perceptual grouping and figure-ground organization. *Psychological Bulletin, 138*, 1172–1217.

Walentynowicz, M., Bogaerts, K., Van Diest, I., Raes, F., & Van den Bergh, O. (2015). Was it so bad? The role of retrospective memory in symptom reporting. *Health Psychology*, *34*, 1166–1174.

Walker, P. (2016). Cross-sensory correspondences and symbolism in spoken and written language. *Journal of Experimental Psychology: Learning, Memory, and Cognition*, *42*, 1339–1361.

Walther, D. B., & Shen, D. (2014). Nonaccidental properties underlie human categorization of complex natural scenes. *Psychological Science*, *25*, 851–860.

Wang, H. X., & Movshon, J. A. (2016). Properties of pattern and component directive-selective cells in area MT of the macaque. *Journal of Neurophysiology*, *115*, 2705–2720.

Wang, J. Y., Zhang, H. T., Chang, J. Y., Woodward, D. J., Baccala, L. A., & Luo, F. (2008). Anticipation of pain enhances the nocioceptive transmission and functional connectivity of within pain network in rats. *Molecular Pain*, *4*. doi:10.1186/1744-8069.

Wang, L., Long, D., Li, Z., & Armour, C. (2011). Posttraumatic stress disorder symptom structure in Chinese adolescents exposed to a deadly earthquake. *Journal of Abnormal Child Psychology*, *39*, 749–758.

Wang, Q. (2004). The emergence of cultural self-constructs. *Developmental Psychology*, *40*, 3–15.

Wang, Q. J., Wang, S., & Spence, C. (2016). "Turn up the taste": Assessing the role of taste intensity and emotion in mediating crossmodal correspondences between basic tastes and pitch. *Chemical Senses*, *41*, 345–356.

Waxman, S. R., & Braun, I. (2005). Consistent (but not variable) names as invitations to form object categories. *Cognition*, *95*, 1359–1368.

Weidemann, G., Satkunarajah, M., & Lovibond, P. F. (2016). I think, therefore eyeblink: The importance of contingency awareness in conditioning. *Psychological Science*, *27*, 467–475.

Weinberger, D. R., & Radulescu, E. (2016). Finding the elusive psychiatric "lesion" with 21st-century neuroanatomy: A note of caution. *American Journal of Psychiatry, 173*, 27–33.

Weissman, M. M., Berry, O. O., Warner, V., Gameroff, M. J., Skipper, J., Talati, A., et al. (2016). A 30-year study of 3 generations at high risk and low risk for depression. *JAMA Psychiatry, 73*, 970–977.

Weisz, G. M. (2015). Secondary guilt syndrome may have led Nazi-persecuted Jewish writers to suicide. *Ramban Maimonides Medical Journal, 26*. doi:10.5041.

Wellman, L. L., Forcelli, P. A., Aguilar, B. L., & Malkova, L. (2016). Bidirectional control of social behavior by activity within basolateral and central amygdala of primates. *Journal of Neuroscience, 36*, 8746–8756.

Wendt, J., Schmidt, L. E., Lotze, M., & Hamm, A. O. (2012). Mechanisms of change: Effects of repetitive exposure to feared stimuli on the brain's fear network. *Psychophysiology, 49*, 1319–1329.

Werner, E., & Smith, R. S. (1982). *Vulnerable but invincible*. New York: McGraw Hill.

Wetzel, N., Buttelmann, D., Schieler, A., & Widmann, A. (2016). Infant and adult pupil dilation in response to unexpected sounds. *Developmental Psychobiology, 58*, 382–392.

Whalen, P. J., Kagan, J., Cook, R. G., Davis, F. C., Kim, H., Polis, S., et al. (2004). Human amygdala responsivity to masked fearful eye whites. *Science, 306*, 2061.

Wheelan, C. (2013). *Naked statistics*. New York: W. W. Norton.

Wiener, K., & Kagan, J. (1976). Infants' reaction to changes in orientation of figure and frame. *Perception, 5*, 25–28.

Wierzbicka, A. (1991). Japanese key words and core cultural values. *Language in Society, 20*, 333–385.

Wierzbicka, A. (1999). *Emotions across languages and cultures*. New York: Cambridge University Press.

Wiggert, N., Wilhelm, F. H., Reichenberger, J., & Blechert, J. (2015). Exposure to social-evaluative video clips: Neural, facial-muscular, and experiential responses and the role of social anxiety. *Biological Psychology*, *110*, 59–67.

Willander, J., & Larsson, M. (2006). Smell your way back to childhood. *Psychonomic Bulletin & Review*, *13*, 240–244.

Willems, R. M., Frank, S. L., Nijhof, A. D., Hagoort, P., & van den Bosch, A. (2016). Prediction during natural language comprehension. *Cerebral Cortex*, *26*, 2506–2516.

Williams, L. E., Oler, J. A., Fox, A. S., McFarlin, D. R., Rogers, G. M., Jesson, M. A., et al. (2015). Fear of the unknown. *Neuropsychopharmacology*, *40*, 1428–1435.

Willmers, C. (2001). *Antonyms in context*. Lund, Sweden: Lund University Press.

Winterer, G., Carver, F. W., Mussa, F., Mattay, V., Weinberger, D. R., & Coppola, R. (2007). Complex relationship between BOLD signal and synchronization/desynchronization of human brain MEG oscillations. *Human Brain Mapping*, *28*, 805–816.

Wise, N. J., Frangos, E., & Komisaruk, B. R. (2016). Activation of sensory cortex by imagined genital stimulation. *Socioaffective Neuroscience & Psychology*, *6*, 31481.

Wojcik, S. P., Hovasapian, A., Graham, J., Motyl, M., & Ditto, P. H. (2015). Conservatives report, but liberal display, greater happiness. *Science*, *347*, 1243–1246.

Wood, D., & Furr, R. M. (2016). The correlates of similarity estimates are often misleading positive. *Personality and Social Psychology Review*, *20*, 79–99.

Woolgar, A., Jackson, J., & Duncan, J. (2016). Coding of visual, auditory, rule, and response information in the brain. *Journal of Cognitive Neuroscience*, *28*, 1433–1454.

Woolston, C. (2016). Group dynamics: A lab of their own. *Nature, 531,* 263–265.

Wright, S. K. (2006). Phonological cues influence sex decisions about novel names. *Psychological Reports, 99,* 315–321.

Xu, Y., & Chun, M. M. (2007). Visual grouping in human parietal cortex. *Proceedings of the National Academy of Sciences of the United States of America, 104,* 18766–18771.

Yanai, I., & Lercher, M. (2016). *The society of genes.* Cambridge, MA: Harvard University Press.

Yoshida, K. C. S., Van Meter, P. E., & Holekamp, K. E. (2016). Variation among free-living spotted hyenas in three personality traits. *Behaviour, 153.* doi:10.1163/1568539x-0003367.

Yoshida, W., Seymour, B., Koltzenburg, M., & Dolan, R. J. (2013). Uncertainty increases pain. *Journal of Neuroscience, 33,* 5638–5646.

Zanto, T. P., Clapp, W. C., Rubens, M. T., Karlsson, J., & Gazzaley, A. (2016). Expectations of task demands dissociate working memory and long-term memory systems. *Cerebral Cortex, 26,* 1176–1186.

Zaytseva, Y., Gutyrchik, E., Bao, Y., Poppel, E., Han, S., Northoff, G., et al. (2014). Self priming in the brain. *Brain and Cognition, 87,* 104–108.

Zentner, M. R., & Kagan, J. (1996). Perception of music by infants. *Nature, 383,* 29.

Zhang, W., Duan, G., Xu, Q., Jia, Z., Bai, Z., Liu, W., et al. (2015). A cross-sectional study on posttraumatic stress disorder and general psychiatric morbidity among adult survivors 3 years after the Wenchuan earthquake, China. *Asia-Pacific Journal of Public Health, 27,* 860–870.

Zhu, D. C., Tarumi, T., Khan, M. A., & Zhang, R. (2015). Vascular coupling in resting-state fMRI: Evidence from multiple modalities. *Journal of Cerebral Blood Flow and Metabolism, 35,* 1910–1920.

Zhu, J., Manichaikul, A., Hu, Y., Chen, Y. I., Liang, S., Steffen, L. M., et al. (2016). Meta-analysis of genome-wide association studies identifies three novel loci for saturated fatty acids in East Asians. *European Journal of Nutrition*, 1–8.

Zijlema, W., Klijs, B., Stolk, R. P., & Rosmalen, J. G. M. (2015). (Un) health in the city. *PLoS One*, *10*, e0143910.

Zlatkina, V., & Petrides, M. (2014). Morphological patterns of the intra-parietal sulcus and the anterior parietal sulcus of Jensen in the human brain. *Proceedings of the Royal Biological Sciences of the Royal Society*, *281*, 1797–1803.

Index